MATH ATTACK:
Strategies for winning the Pharmacology Math Battle

MATH ATTACK:
Strategies for winning the Pharmacology Math Battle

Karen Stuart Champion RN, MS

Nursethings
Fort Pierce, FL 34982

Notice to the Reader:

ISBN13: 978-0-9759998-5-1
ISBN: 0-9759998-5-0

Nursethings
www.nursethings.com

Table of Contents

Introduction

Pharmacology math seems to strike fear in the hearts of nursing students. It needn't be that way. This book takes a completely different approach to solving pharmacology math problems than other books I have seen. It is based on a method I have used to help countless students go from failing math tests to acing them. Surprisingly it is not about the math skills. It is about making sense of it all, figuring out where to start and confidence. This book will help you understand the meaning of questions, pitfalls to watch out for, and formulas to use. You CAN win the battle, I am sure of it!

☺ Karen Champion

1 ✳ Why Does Pharmacology Math Seem So Difficult? ✳ 1

Nothing seems to put more fear into a nursing student than pharmacology math tests. From the very beginning of the nursing program all the way until the final semester the math tests cause most students stress. Students use words such as anxiety, hysteria, panic, and sheer terror to describe their state of mind before math tests.

If pharmacology math is such torture why do it?

Math is a necessary component of nursing care. It is still necessary to calculate some medication dosages and infuse fluids by calculating the flow rate. Medication errors make up about 10% of fatal medical errors so regardless of your feelings pharmacology math is serious business. Because the nurse is the person usually administering the medication they are the last chance to prevent errors. Pharmacology math tests don't end with nursing school either. It is standard procedure to take a pharmacology math test and pass it before being hired for any nursing job. So you must mend your relationship with math or forever be haunted by it.

The good news is that I have yet to meet a student that could not master pharmacology math after working with me. In fact some students referred to me were on their last chance to pass the test or had even dropped out and started over. After spending two hours with me and the process laid out in this book these students have gone on to be successful in math. These were good students and have gone on to be great nurses and you can do it too! You can enjoy the challenge of pharmacology math!

What makes pharmacology math hard?

✳ Your nursing instructor might hate math too!

You might be surprised to find out that your nursing instructor teaching you how to do these calculations may only know one way to do the calculations and may not really understand how to explain how it works. It was the one way they learned it and so the cycle continues. Have you noticed a lot of nursing programs simply tell you to buy the book and learn it on your own or if you mention an alternate method look at you with that deer in the headlights stare.

✳ Calculation problems are word problems

Even math teachers aren't too hip on word problems. Mixing words and numbers isn't easy for anyone. In pharmacology math it is made more difficult be adding in words and abbreviations that you have never heard of and may not understand yet. Because it is difficult to understand the context even math instructors have a hard time.

✳ Calculating and Touch-Feely don't usually go together

The personality or cognitive make up of people drawn to nursing may be less mathematically oriented. If you have ever done a personality profile or something that looks at left brain versus right brain it is interesting that math heavy jobs such as accounting and engineering are frequently mirror opposites of nurses and social workers. It is not a gender thing either.

❋ High school may have been a long time ago and simple algebra was never really that simple.

If you don't like math I doubt you are entering nursing after a successful career as an accountant. So you may have been avoiding math all these years. It may be like riding a bike—it comes back to you eventually but it may feel like you learned on a tricycle and now they're asking you to mountain bike down Pike's Peak. Guess what? Even students who have just successfully completed college algebra have difficulties with this. That is really heartbreaking. Some female students may have been brainwashed that girls aren't good in math or like math. Male students may feel really bad if they are having problems because after all they are supposed to be good in math. Both assumptions are absolutely false. Younger students hopefully haven't been exposed to those stereotypes. There are also some common problem areas or math pitfalls as I call them that you need to keep in mind **(Chapter 3)**.

❋ The word math makes you have palpitations and break out in a cold sweat

Math anxiety is nothing new. There are even math teachers who have done dissertations on math anxiety, worked tirelessly to end math anxiety, and spent late nights trying to come up with methods to help students. I won't go into the body of research on the subject because most can be helped quite a bit with simple methods. However, if you have an extreme case of math anxiety know that you are not the only one and help is out there. I suggest trying the techniques in this book and if they do not help then check other resources available at your school and do a search on the internet for math anxiety.

Reducing anxiety surrounding pharmacology math

1. **Learn the language (Chapter 2)**—If you don't know the terminology, measurement systems, or abbreviations the questions are going to look like they are written in a foreign language. There is no way around the fact that you must memorize this information as soon as possible. Making and using flashcards is an easy and portable way to accomplish this task.

2. **Controlled breathing**—Slowly inhale and exhale 5 times before you get started. Focusing on that physical act helps distract you from your anxiety

3. **Positive Mantra**—Ever notice when you are about to do something you aren't confident about you hear messages in your head that seem to seem to become self fulfilling prophecies? Such as "I can't do this", "Oh I suck at math", or 'I don't know what I am doing". Develop some positive statements to help put you in a good frame of mind such as "I am a good problem solver", "I am successful at math" or even acknowledging your feelings "I am fearful of making an error so I will do my best to be accurate".

4. **Earplugs**—OK not such a good suggestion for clinical but when taking a test earplugs help to block out the distractions of rustling papers, erasing, and people moving around. This is useful for any exam especially for auditory learners that are especially prone to distraction from classroom noise. In clinical be sure to step away to a quiet place to do your calculations and always check them with your instructor.

5. **Self-Direction**—This helps you focus on one step at a time rather than the whole problem, which can be overwhelming and self-defeating. So when you are looking at a problem and you start thinking "where do I even begin?" give yourself directions in your head to get started such as "First I need to determine if a calculation is needed...Next I will..." and so on. Which leads us to ...

6. **Use a structured step-by-step approach**—Do I dare say that you already can do this math? Yes that's right you don't need this book to show you how to multiply, divide and so on. What makes my method different from other books is it gives you a step-by-step approach to the problems and how to figure out what formula to use. All of your basic problems can be approached the same way and you only need two formulas. The **Math Scaffold (Chapter 4)** helps you get started. This streamlined approach helps you always know what formula to use and be successful at many different types of problems.

7. **PRACTICE, PRACTICE, PRACTICE!!!**—This really speaks for itself. The more you practice the more confident and comfortable you will be with the calculations. Think about it like any other skill you learn in nursing school. Which student would be the most competent at performing a procedure? A) The student who has looked at the procedure in the book, B) The student that has performed the procedure once in the lab or C) The student that has performed the procedure 100 times in the lab. I am pretty sure the answer is "C". Practice helps to build confidence and help you isolate what kinds of problems are giving you the most trouble. Make sure you take a few minutes each semester to do a couple practice problems to keep it fresh you never know when it will come up next.

Note about examples and answers

Worked out examples and answers to practice problems show individual steps and have equations rewritten so that each step can be understood. When actually doing a problem it is not necessary to do this. The additional practice section only contains the actual answers mainly to save space. However one of the best ways to work on additional problems is to refer to the worked out examples. But I won't leave you hanging if you can't figure out how to get the answer. Simply email your question to me at Karen@nursethings.com and I will work the problem out with the formula you like and can either fax or email it back to you. In fact I would be glad to do this for any pharmacology math question that you come across and for which you need help even if it is not from my book.

2 ✳ Learning the Language ✳ 2

There will be many words, abbreviations, and even some measurements in nursing that will be new to you. Face it you are going to learn a whole new language. Making and using flashcards will help you memorize the necessities fast so you can get on to the fun part of learning a new language such as calling your brother a "bezoar" or scoring big time in scrabble with "zygomaticoauricularis". On a serious note you could figure out why Doctors name all the really heinous diseases after themselves, I have always wondered about that. Okay back to what you need to know to decipher what a medication order is telling you

Anatomy of a medication order

A medication order has certain required components in order for it to be valid. It must have the drug name, dose, route, and time / interval. In the clinical setting remember it must also be signed by a health care provider to be valid. Because errors can cause serious problems for patients the allowed abbreviations are changing. Be sure to check out the warning section at the end of this chapter and any policies in place at the facilities you go to for clinical.

Drug name

Suffice it to say there are a lot of drug names. Individual drugs may even have several names. At the very least there is usually a chemical name, a generic name, and a trade name. While there are only one chemical name and one generic for each drug there may be several trade or "brand" names. You are not gong to be able to memorize all these names but you should be able to look them up in a reference and the order should be written clearly so that you can tell what it is. For pharmacology math it does not matter what the name of the drug is, if you could pronounce it, or what it's used for so don't get hung up on the name.

Drug dose

The drug dose will consist of a number and a measurement qualifier. Here's where the measurement systems and their abbreviations come into play. The three systems of measurement seen on calculation tests are metric, apothecary, and household. In clinical almost everything is in a metric measurement or a measurement unique to the medication such as a "unit" or milliequivalent. Let's start out with those items to get them out of the way.

Unit—an agreed upon standard of measurement of an individual drug. A unit of "drug A" is not equivalent to anything but a unit of "drug A". Two very important drugs that you will use frequently are measured in units, insulin and heparin. Insulin "units" and heparin "units" are not equivalent in volume or any other way.

Millequivalent—This measurement has to do with electrolytes in solution. Because it has to do with the valence and molecular weight of the electrolyte and those items are different for different electrolytes a mEq of potassium is only equivalent to a mEq of potassium.

Measurements and Abbreviations to learn for Pharmacology Math

Metric	Apothecary	Household /Misc.
Kilogram (kg) Gram (g) Milligram (mg) Microgram (mcg or µg) Liter (l or L) Milliliter (ml) (Cubic centimeter (cc))	Grains (gr) (Drams dr) (Minims m) (Scruple)	Pound (lb) Fluid ounce (oz.) Tablespoon (Tb) Teaspoon (tsp) Cup

Items in parentheses should not be used in orders. Grains is rarely used and may be added to the do not use list soon.

Equivalents

Metric
1000 grams   = 1 Kilogram
1000 milligrams   = 1 gram
1000 micrograms   = 1 milligram

1000 milliliter   = 1 Liter
1 milliliter   = 1 cubic centimeter
Note: "cc" is **not recommended for use** in med orders because of risk of misinterpretation and error

Additional important metric equivalent that's not important for drug calculations
1 kilogram = 1 liter of water. This is important for patients that you are concerned about being fluid overloaded. Sudden weight changes indicate fluid changes. So for example a patient has a weight increase of 5 lbs in one day (a little more than 2 kg) they have retained 2 liters of fluid.

Equivalents between Systems

1 Kilogram   = 2.2 pounds
1 grain   = 60 mg (some texts say 62.5 or 65 there is a 10% leeway)
1 fluid ounce   = 30ml
1 cup   = 8 ounces = 240 mlliliters
1 teaspoon   = 5 milliliters
1 tablespoon   = 15 mlliliters

Just for curiosity sake:
1 scruple = 20 grains (Didn't you always wonder what a scruple was equivalent to?)
60 grains = 1 dram = 60 minums
8 drams = 1ounce
Truthfully in 20 years in nursing I haven't seen a dram or minim and fortunately just an occasional lack of scruples.

Route and Time / Interval Abbreviations

The route is how the medication will get into the patients body. Time / Interval is when or how often the patient will receive the medication. There may be other instructions or parameters in the order to give more specific information about when to give or hold the medication. For not recommended abbreviations the term should simply be written out.

Abbreviation / Meaning

ā   before

ac   before meals

ad lib   as desired

AU, AS, AD   Both ear, Left ear, and R ear **(not recommended for use)**

BID   twice a day

c̄   With

D/C   Discontinue **(not recommended for use)**

DS   Double strength

H, hr   hour

HS   hour of sleep, give at bedtime

(HS can mean half strength but **not recommended for use)**

IM   intramuscular injection

IU   International Unit **(not recommended for use)**

IV   intravenous

IVPB   intravenous piggyback, indicates intermittent infusion

μg   Microgram **(not recommended for use)**

Neb   nebulized

NGT   nasogastric tube

NPO   nothing per os (mouth)

OU, OS, OD   Both eye , Left eye, and R eye **(not recommended for use)**

PEG or G-tube   types of gastric access tube

p̄   After

pc   After meals

prn   when needed

q   each /every

Q AM   each morning

QD   Every day **(not recommended for use)**

Q2H   Every 2 hours   Q4H   Every 4 hours   Q6H   Every 6 hours

Q8H   Every 8 hours   Q12H   Every 12 hours   Q24H   Every 24 hours

QHS   Every night before bed (hour of sleep)

QID   Four times a day

QOD   Every other day **(not recommended for use)**

s̄   Without

SC or SQ   Subcutaneous **(not recommended for use)**

SL   Sublingual

SR   Sustained release

STAT   Give Immediately

Supp   suppository

Susp   Suspension

Tab   Tablet

TID   Three times a day

Top   topical

U   units **(not recommended for use)**

XL   Sustained release

Why are there so many "Not recommended for use"?

In recent years there has been more research into medical errors and their root causes. Misinterpretations of abbreviations in written orders have led to many medication errors. Many agencies and organizations have concerns and work together in the **National Coordinating Council for Medication Error Reporting and Prevention (www.nccmerp.org)**. Recommendations for accuracy in prescription writing and a list of dangerous abbreviations with errors associated with them can be found on their website. JCAHO, the Joint Commission on the Accreditation of Healthcare Organizations even has a DO NOT USE list of abbreviations available on its website www.jcaho.org. Check out these great websites for information about preventing medication errors. Why did I include the abbreviations even if they aren't recommended for use? Well unless your instructor has updated their calculation exams very recently you will still see these abbreviations. You may see some in clinical although that seems to be changing pretty quickly.

Examples of medication orders and what they mean

Order	Meaning
Benadryl 50 mg PO Q6H prn itching	The patient can have 50 mg of the drug Benadryl every six hours as needed for itching
Ancef 1 gram IVPB now	Infuse a little bag that contains 1 gram of the drug Ancef intravenously
D5W at 60 ml/hr	Start a continuous intravenous infusion of the solution Dextrose 5% in water to infuse 60 ml into the patient each hour
Heparin 5,000 units, SQ Q12H	Inject 5000 units of the drug heparin into the patient's subcutaneous layer every 12 hours
Metoprolol 12.5 mg PO Daily hold for SBP less than 100	Give the patient 12.5 mg of the drug metoprolol every day but hold it (don't give it) if the systolic (top number) of their blood pressure is less than 100 mmHg
Demerol 50 mg IM Q4H prn pain	Inject 50 mg of the drug Demerol into the patient's muscle every 4 hours if the patient is having pain and needs it

3 ✳ Math Pitfalls ✳ 3

This section consists of areas students have forgotten since they last had a math class or seem to consistently have difficulty with and peculiarity of pharmacology math.

Order of Operations

This is not the OR schedule for the day it is the agreed upon order of proceeding with computations when there is more than one kind of operation to be performed. Unlike extreme makeover where it probably doesn't matter if they lipo the thighs then the stomach or vice versa in math not following the correct order will cause you to come up with incorrect answers.

The accepted order is as follows: Parenthesis, exponents, multiply, divide, add, subtract. When faced with doing more than one operation at a time you must follow the order of operations.

Now fortunately pharmacology math doesn't involve exponents. In fact the problems we face are actually not very complex and all you really need to remember is to **multiply then divide**! There may only be small differences if you divide first but it will give you odd decimals where there should be whole numbers (which may or may not be acceptable to your instructor).

Issues with Decimals

You must be extra careful with decimals. A mistake of one decimal place means a ten-fold difference in the answer. Ten times the dose of many medications can be fatal, that's right fatal as in dead! Medications that involve decimals usually involve small quantities of high potency medications. Definitely double check your calculations and write it out long hand. When you multiply remember to put all the decimal places combined of the numbers multiplied back in and when you divide move the decimals over so you are dividing with a whole number. It's a good idea to go ahead and put the decimal where it belongs before dividing.

$$\begin{array}{r} 12.5 \\ \underline{3.2} \\ 250 \\ \underline{375} \\ 40.00 \end{array}$$

There are two decimal places in the numbers being multiplied

So you must put the same amount back into the answer

$$0.125\overline{\smash{)}0.25}$$

$$0.125\overline{\smash{)}0.250}$$

$$125\overline{\smash{)}250}$$

You need to divide by a whole number. So in order to do that you must move the decimal over three spots in the divisor (0.125) and the dividend (0.25). This is equivalent to multiplying both sides of the equation by 1000. Put the decimal on top so it will already be in the correct place for your answer.

Issues with Fractions

Fractions can be quit scary for people but it doesn't have to be. There are only a few things to remember about fractions for pharmacology math.

A fraction is made up of two parts a numerator (the **n**umber on top) and the denominator (demons live down below). A fraction means the numerator divided by the denominator.

This number $\Longrightarrow$ <u>Numerator</u> such as $\dfrac{2}{4}$
Divided by this number $\Longrightarrow$ Denominator

When you multiply fractions you multiple across meaning the numerators are multiplied then the denominators. In keeping with order of operations you multiply then divide.

Remember a whole number really has a denominator of 1 but we don't write it that way because its unnecessary. If there is no denominator it is known and accepted that it is a whole number. However it is important to remember this fact when you are multiplying a fraction times a whole number so that you multiply the correct numbers together.

This is especially important when there is a fraction within a fraction

$$\frac{\frac{1}{2}}{4} \times 6 =$$

$$\frac{\frac{1}{2} \times \frac{6}{1}}{4} = \frac{\frac{6}{2}}{4} = \frac{3}{4}$$ You must multiply numerator with numerator

$$\frac{\frac{1}{2}}{4} \times 6 \neq \frac{\frac{1}{12}}{4}$$ Common error is to multiple the denominator with the numerator

Reducing fractions will help make the math easier if you don't have a calculator and are dealing with big numbers.

$$\frac{5}{25} = \frac{1}{5} \times \frac{5}{5} \qquad \frac{5}{5} = 1 \qquad 5\overline{)\frac{1}{5}}$$ Because the numerator and denominator are both divisible by 5 they can both be reduced and because 5 divided by 5 is equal to one it is equivalent to the original fraction

$$\frac{10}{40} \times 8$$ You can reduce more than once but you can only reduce one numerator with one denominator at a time.

$$\frac{10}{40} \times 8 \qquad \frac{1}{4} \times \frac{8^2}{1} = 2$$

$$\frac{10}{40} \times \frac{8^1}{1} \qquad \frac{2\,10}{1\,8} \times \frac{P}{1} = 2$$ 10 was divided out of 10 and the 40 then 4 was divided out of the 4 and 8, that's okay. Next row 8 was divided out of the 8 and the 40 then 5 was divided out of 10 and the 5, that's okay.

$$\frac{10}{40} \times 8 \neq \frac{5}{20} \times 4$$ In this example 2 was divided out of the 10, 40, and 8 all at once this is NOT okay

Solving for X Concepts

The key to solving for "X" is to get "X" by itself then you have your answer. "X" = _____ In the formulas that have an "X" the only thing you will have to do is divide both sides by the coefficient of "X". The coefficient is simply the number multiplied by "X". To be fair and mathematically correct you must divide both sides by that number or it won't work out. What you do to one side of an equation you must do to the other in terms of operations. If the coefficient is a fraction you multiple each side by the denominator to get rid of the denominator.

Rounding in drug calculations

In pharmacology math you mostly use regular rounding rules with a major consideration. You only round if you can't administer the amount of your answer. For example you can give 0.5 tablets in fact rounding 0.5 to 1 would be giving the patient twice the ordered dose which is not acceptable. But in the case of a gtts/min answer of 20.66 you cannot deliver .66 of a drop it is impossible. So you would round your answer to 21. Syringes come in many sizes. Medications for injection can be given in amounts to 2 decimal places if less than a milliliter and to one decimal place in larger syringes. So it is possible to give 0.75 ml and 2.5 ml. You would not round up those answers because you can administer that exact amount. Because you have to learn this math usually before you have even seen syringes or know what IV tubing looks like take the time to go to your nursing lab and look at some. At the very least look at the pictures in your fundamentals text so you have some context for your rounding decisions.

½ Tab or 2 tabs Big Difference!

When the dose ordered or on hand is twice the other it looks like a super easy, do it in your head calculation but BE CAREFUL! If you give ½ when you should be giving 2 tablets that is only ¼ of the dose and if you give 2 tablets that's 4 times the ordered dose. With some medications that could be fatal. Be safe and do the math!

Using calculators

You may or may not be allowed to use calculators on exams. You may or may not have one available in clinical the day you need one. My advice is to do the math long hand using your brain. If you have difficulty with the basic multiplication and division required for these calculations you are in serious need of math remediation. Look for resources at your school or in your community which are usually free to help you. While you may like using a calculator and it may make things faster be sure its used for convenience not to because you can't actually do the math.

Your calculator only does what you tell it to do. If you put things into the calculator in an incorrect manner it will give you an answer that is incorrect. Math phobic people tend to believe the calculator is smarter than they are but that is not true. Depending on the complexity of your calculator and the type of formula you are using putting in your information may be different. A basic calculator from the dollar store works just fine but remember your order of operations

Say you have this fraction to solve: $\frac{9 \times 8 \times 4}{3 \times 2}$

You put it in the calculator as follows:

9x8x4 / 3x2 = 192 Moving left to right the calculator is faced with one operation at a time so it does the calculations as 9 multiplied by 8 = 72 multiplied by 4 = 288 divided by 3 = 96 multiplied by 2 equals192 This isn't correct.

In your original problem 3x2 is the denominator so it should be either in parentheses if your calculator does that or multiplied separately before dividing. Remember if there are two things to do the calculator will follow the order of operations and multiply what is in the parentheses first then divide. You could put the numerator in its own parentheses as well but in this case it isn't necessary.
9*8*4 / (3*2) = 48 Inputted in this way the calculator does the calculations as 9 multiplied by 8 = 72 multiplied by4 = 288 divided by the outcome of 3x2.

If your calculator does not have parentheses you will have to put in 9x8x4= 288 and write that down then 3x2=6 Next do 288 / 6 = 48.

Cruel and Unusual

I hate to even bring this up but sometimes there are cruel and unusual problems on math tests. Some are there because the test hasn't been updated since 1965. Some are there because nurses have a hard time of letting go of the past. Some are just poorly written questions. I can't fully explain or justify why some of these questions persist.

＊ Questions using outdated forms of measurement. If you come across an order written in minims in clinical it would be highly unusual as I have never seen one in 20 years of nursing. Okay you will have to learn grains. That continues to be a hanger on-ner but fortunately its not really used in real life either. Maybe it's the old "I had to learn it so you do too"

＊ Questions where the correct answer is not a real amount you would give a patient. Imagine you have heard how serious a med error is and you come up with an answer of 84 tablets on question 2 of your exam. In good conscious you are going to make yourself crazy trying to figure that out because you know 84 tablets can't possibly be the answer. You get it wrong when you break down and put 2 for the answer.

＊ Questions that give you the answer and require you to work backwards. Such as: you assess a patient's IV dripping at 20 gtts/min with a 10 gtt set, what is the patient's hourly rate? I have to say I am morally opposed to questions like these because absolutely no nurse goes into a patient's room and does this. On the other hand if you can do this math backwards in addition to forwards you are pretty good. Most likely your teacher copied the question from a test bank without really looking at it and won't be to eager to explain how or when this procedure is done. Enough ranting already. Here is how you would solve this question. The piece of information you usually have but don't this time becomes "X" and you fill everything in where it fits in the formula. So it is a basic solve for "X" problem.

$$\frac{X}{60} \times 10 = 20 \text{ gtts/min}$$ Fill everything in

$$(60)\frac{X}{60} \times 10 = 20\,(60)$$ Multiply both sides of the equation by 60, we are working to get "X" by itself

$$\cancel{(60)}\frac{X}{\cancel{60}} \times 10 = 1200$$ The 60's cancel out on the left

$$10X = 1200$$ Next "X" x 10 is the same as 10X

$$\frac{\cancel{10}}{\cancel{10}}X = \frac{120\cancel{0}}{1\cancel{0}}$$ Divide both sides by 10 again in our quest to get "X" by itself

$$X = 120 \text{ ml/hr}$$ Finally the answer.

✱ Questions where the on hand is in outdated measurement systems such as grains. These questions are solved just like any other conversion questions but because grains are expressed as fractions and you will end up dividing fractions it is a headache. The good news is you will never see this in real life.

Ordered: Morphine 10 mg IM Q4H prn pain
On Hand: Morphine gr ¼ / oz

$10\,mg : gr\,X = 60\,mg : gr\,1$

$60x = 10$

$\frac{60}{60}x = \frac{10}{60}$

$x = \frac{1}{6}$

$gr\,\frac{1}{6} : X\,oz : gr\,\frac{1}{4} : 1\,oz$

$\frac{1}{4}x = \frac{1}{6}$

$(4)\frac{1}{4}x = \frac{1}{6}(4)$

$x = \frac{4}{6} \ or \ \frac{2}{3}\,oz$

Ratio Proportion

$\dfrac{10\,mg}{gr\,X} \diagtimes \dfrac{60\,mg}{gr\,1}$

$60x = 10$

$\frac{60}{60}x = \frac{10}{60}$

$x = gr\,\frac{1}{6}$

$\dfrac{gr\,\frac{1}{6}}{X\,oz} \diagtimes \dfrac{gr\,\frac{1}{4}}{1\,oz}$

$\frac{1}{4}x = \frac{1}{6}$

$(4)\frac{1}{4}x = \frac{1}{6}(4)$

$x = \frac{4}{6} \ or \ \frac{2}{3}\,oz$

Fraction Method

$\dfrac{10\,mg}{60\,mg} \times gr\,1 = \frac{1}{6}$

$\dfrac{gr\,\frac{1}{6}}{gr\,\frac{1}{4}} \times 1\,oz = \frac{1}{6} \overset{\to 4}{\times} \frac{}{\to 1} = \frac{4}{6}$

$= \frac{2}{3}\,oz$

Desired over Have

$10\,mg \times \dfrac{gr\,1}{60\,mg} \times \dfrac{1\,oz}{gr\,\frac{1}{4}} = \dfrac{\frac{10}{60}}{\frac{1}{4}} = \frac{10}{15} = \frac{2}{3}\,oz$

Dimensional Analysis

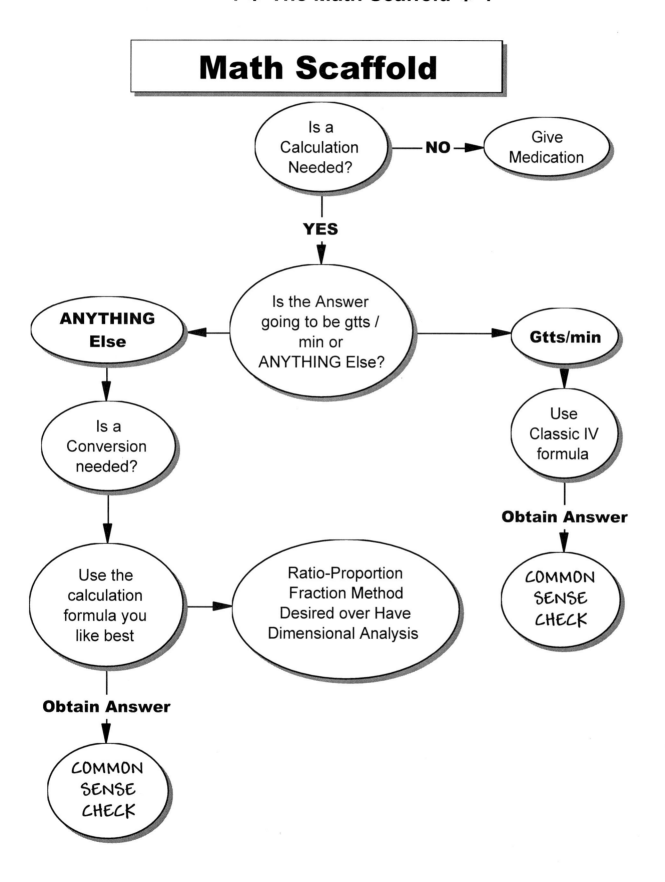

The **Math Scaffold** is a road map of what to do given any problem. It gives you a starting point. It is really a thought process on paper. There is an extra copy of the math scaffold in the answer section in the back of the book if you want to tear one out to have in front of you when you are doing practice problems. Let us go through the math scaffold level by level.

First, **"Is a calculation needed?"** If you are taking a "calculation test" the answer to this question is likely to be yes. In clinical it may be yes or no. Why start with such a simple question? It gets you started!

Next, **"Is the answer going to be gtts/min (drops per minute) or ANYTHING ELSE?"** If the answer is going to be <u>gtts /min</u> you take the path on the right if the answer is going to be <u>anything else</u>, which could be tablets, mg, ml/hr, ml, capsules...anything besides gtts/min you will take the left path.

Following the right path you will use the classic IV formula to calculate your answer. It's the simplest way to calculate gtts/min.

Following the left path **"Is a conversion is needed"** is next. This is not scary it is a yes or no question. It doesn't necessarily make solving the overall question more difficult it just means you will have two calculations if you like using one of the first three formulas or have an additional part to the calculation if you choose the last formula. Let's stay with the question at hand "Is a conversion needed" for the moment. This is an easy question to answer by looking at the qualifiers. If there are more than two different qualifiers you will need to do a conversion. You will need to convert what's ordered to the form of measurement of what is on hand. For example:

Ordered: happypill 0.2 g, PO, QD
On hand: happypill 400 mg tablets

You have three different qualifiers—g, mg, and tablets. A conversion is needed. To do a conversion you will need to know the conversion factor. Conversion factors are simply equivalents between measurements that you will just have to memorize such as 1 g = 1,000 mg. Common conversion factors you will need for pharmacology math are listed in Chapter 2.

Ordered: happypill 200 mg, PO, QD
On hand: happypill 400 mg tablets

You have only two different qualifiers—mg, mg and tablets. No conversion is needed because the ordered amount is in mg and the on hand amount is in mg.

Once you know if a conversion is needed (simply yes or no at this point) you move on to **"Use the calculation formula you like best"** You probably don't like any of them at this point (or even know what they are) don't worry they grow on you. If no conversion is needed you will use one formula one time. If a conversion is needed you will use one formula twice if you like ratio-proportion, fraction, or desired over have. With dimensional analysis you will add a step into the single formula.

The math scaffold says **"Use the calculation formula you like best"** You only need one formula when your answer is "anything else". It will work for everything where the answer is anything other than gtts / min. Its not a choice of having a formula but you do have a choice of which one. Believe me instructors get nervous when a student is not sure what formula they used and aren't sure how they got that answer. The other benefit for finding the one formula that works best for you and using it every time is that doing it the same way each time provides consistency, builds confidence, and improves competence. Different formulas appeal to different people. You need to give all four a try and pick which one works the best for you. Once you have chosen a formula you can completely ignore, forget, or otherwise have nothing to do with the others. In the following pages there are explanations of each of the formulas with examples. You are then asked to do ten problems using all four methods. This is a very important process. Once you have completed the problems you will likely have a feeling of which formula works best for you. Now that you have a formula for "everything else" all you have left to learn is the classic IV formula and you are ready to tackle the practice problems and any calculation test that comes your way.

My Formula is: _____

(fill in this space once you have completed the selection process)

It was so exciting to find your formula I almost forgot about the final step in the math scaffold **"the common sense step"**. This is vital in preventing errors. It is basically asking your self "does this answer make sense". Some answers will scream math errors. Common sense will tell you that answers such as 84 tablets, 13.4 ml for an injection, 100 ml of an elixir, 650 gtts/min cannot be right. They are so far from a usual dose hopefully you would realize they are not correct. Nursing judgment comes in when the error is less obvious. As you gain more experience this will get easier but in the mean time that is why it is important to look up dosages and consider your patient as an individual. Two tablets of a particular medication may be too much and you may give six tablets of another medication and it is okay. A patient's condition, body weight, renal function etc. may play a role in dosages of medications. As you are starting out I am hoping you have the common sense to identify obvious errors and the common sense to ask when you are not sure.

Other tips to avoid medication errors—Think 1, 2, 3, C, C, C. (From Survival Tips for the Nursing Student in Med-Surg Clinicals)

One
Question giving anything SQ/SC that is greater than 1cc. Most SQ injections are less than 1cc in volume. Greater than 1cc, you should question.

Two
Question giving anything IV push that is greater than 2cc IV push meds can range from 0.1 to 50 cc in volume but *most are 0.5 to 2 cc.* In general question if the volume is >2 cc. Check to see if volume provides a dose that is within normal range.

Question giving more than 2 of the same type of pills. If you are giving more than **2** pills of any kind of medication, ask yourself "IS this an acceptable dosage?" Look it up, ask pharmacy, and if it is not within a normal dose range justification should be noted in the progress notes or the order should be verified with the ordering physician.

Always have 2 nurses check insulin/heparin before administering

Three
Question giving anything IM that is greater than 3cc. Most IM injections are 0.5 to 3cc in volume. Greater than **3cc**, you should question. If the volume is greater than **3cc** more than one injection will be needed to accomplish the dose.

Check Chart

If you are unsure of the medication, dosage, or route always *check the chart* for the original order

Clear Color

Question giving anything IV, IM, SQ that is not clear. Most IV/IM, and SQ meds (not all) are clear. Some exceptions are: some insulins, TPN, Lipids, Diprivan, multivitamin. However, the majority of IV/IM, and SQ medications are clear. It is better to question and get clarification before administration.

Compatibility Chart

Question the compatibility if you are giving two or more things together. Make sure that if you are giving two or more things together whether it be in an IV or in an injection, check for compatibility. There are compatibility charts for both injectable forms and intravenous forms of medication.

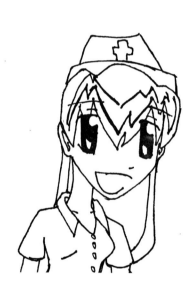

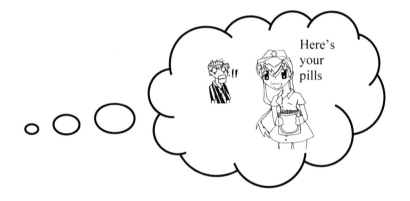

150 tablets would be too many to be correct!

5 ✳ Anything Else Formulas ✳ 5

You have a choice for your "anything else" formula. It is important to use each of the formulas to find which one works best for you. Each formula will give the same answer because they are accomplishing the same task even though they each have a slightly different set-up. Mathematically they are doing the same thing and for this reason you only need one formula to do the job.

The four formulas are:
    Ratio-Proportion
    Fraction Method
    Desired over Have (also called "The Formula")
    Dimensional Analysis

Similarities and Differences, Pros and Cons

Ratio-Proportion and the **Fraction method** are almost identical. The difference is that Ratio-Proportion is lying down and the Fraction method is standing up so to speak. As similar as these two are they attract completely different people. Ratio-Proportion is very linear and sometimes appeals more to linear people. Someone who always starts on page one of the chapter, doesn't skip around, moves from the beginning to the end in a straight line. The fraction method usually appeals to more global, big picture type people who just by liking fractions so much could be considered a bit strange (I can say that because I am in this group myself). Both of these formulas involve solving for an unknown "X". While the "X" is just holding the place of the number you are calculating just the fact it is there freaks out some people.

Desired over Have or as its sometime known "The Formula" is the old time-y method taught to nurses. A lot of nurses like it because there is no "X" in the formula and the name itself implies how to fill in the problem. However, the whole name should be "Desired over Have times the units it comes in". If that last part is not in there you can have an error. While some might consider this formula old school it works just fine and is very close to **Dimensional Analysis.** Dimensional Analysis is like a hybrid Desired over Have. When filling in the formula the focus is on the qualifiers rather than the numbers and you can put any necessary conversions in as you go along. Another great aspect of Dimensional Analysis (besides the intensely intellectual sounding name) is that it is used in other courses to do math problems, in particular chemistry (yet another subject nurses tend to dislike).

With **Ratio-Proportion, Fraction method, and Desired over Have** it will be necessary use the formula twice when there is a conversion. One set up to do the conversion and one to do the drug calculation. With **Dimensional Analysis** the conversion factor is added into the over all problem so everything is done at once. It can make the problem look rather large though and some will find this overwhelming.

6 ✳ Ratio-Proportion ✳ 6

Ratio-Proportion basic structure is:

$$\frac{\text{(cloud)}}{} : \text{(cloud)} = \text{(cloud)} : \text{(cloud)}$$

Once everything is in its place you multiply the means (numbers closest to the equal signs) and the extremes (the ones on the end) and use basic techniques for solving for "X" described in chapter 3.

Because there is an "X" involved it is helpful to use a statement to fill in the blanks. These sound weird at first and will make more sense when used with the examples.

Statement for a conversion: I know that (drug name) (amount) (unit of measurement of what's ordered) is ordered but I don't know (X) how many (units of measurement of what's on hand) that equals, but I do know (conversion factor).

Statement to figure out what is what for a dosage calculation: I know that (drug name) (amount) (unit of measurement / qualifier) is ordered but I don't know how it comes (X). But I do know or I have on hand (drug name) (amount) (unit of measurement / qualifier) comes in (amount / form)

Problem without a conversion example:
 Ordered: Happypill 200 mg, PO, QD
 On hand: Happypill 400 mg tablets

Using the math scaffold: a calculation is needed and the answer is going to be "anything else". No conversion is needed because I only have two different qualifiers, mg and tablets.

Using the statement to fill in the structure:

$$200mg : X tab = 400mg : 1 tab$$

I know that Happypill 200 mg is ordered but I don't know how it comes (X). But I do know Happypill 400 mg comes in one tablet.

IMPORTANT: Notice that mg is in the first position on both sides. This is very important. The qualifier in the first position on each side must match and the qualifier in the second position on each side must match for this to work.

$$200 mg : X tab = 400 mg : 1 tab$$

Now solve by multiplying the means and extremes then solving for "X"

$$400x = 200$$

$$\frac{400X}{400} = \frac{200}{400}$$

Get "X" by itself by dividing both sides by 400

$$X = \frac{2}{4}$$

Reduce to get the final answer

$$X = \frac{1}{2} tab$$

Problem with a conversion example:
  Ordered: Happypill 0.2 g, PO, QD
  On hand: Happypill 400 mg tablets

Using the math scaffold: a calculation is needed and the answer is going to be "anything else". A conversion is needed because I have three different qualifiers g, mg, and tablets.

You can go ahead and draw two formula structures to remind you that there are going to be two calculations

Using the statement for a conversion:

$$0.2g : Xmg = 1g : 1000mg$$

I know that Happypill 0.2 g is ordered but I don't know (X) how many mg that equals, but I do know that 1g equal 1000mg.

IMPORTANT: Notice that g is in the first position on both sides. This is very important. The qualifier in the first position on each side must match and the qualifier in the second position on each side must match for this to work.

$$0.2g : Xmg = 1g : 1000mg$$

$$X = \frac{1000}{0.2}$$

$$200.0$$

$$X = 200mg$$

Now solve by multiplying the means and extremes then solving for "X". To be extra careful if you are calculating by hand you might want to do that calculation on the side to avoid decimal errors.

Now you know that 0.2 g = 200mg, the order is equivalent to Happypill 200mg. PO, QD

Using the math scaffold: a calculation is needed and the answer is going to be "anything else". No conversion is needed because I only have two different qualifiers, mg and tablets.

Using the statement to fill in the structure:

$$200mg : Xtab = 400mg : 1 tab$$

I know that Happypill 200 mg is ordered but I don't know how it comes (X). But I do know Happypill 400 mg comes in one tablet.

$$200mg : Xtab = 400mg : 1tab$$

$$400x = 200$$

$$\frac{400X}{400} = \frac{200}{400}$$

Now solve by multiplying the means and extremes then solving for "X"

Get "X" by itself by dividing both sides by 400

$$X = \frac{2}{4}$$

$$X = \frac{1}{2} tab$$

Reduce to get the final answer

19

7 ✳ Fraction Method ✳ 7

Fraction Method basic structure is:

Once everything is in its place you cross-multiply and use basic techniques for solving for "X" described in chapter 3. Because there is an "X" involved it is helpful to use a statement to fill in the blanks. These sound weird at first and will make more sense when used with the examples.

Statement for a conversion: I know that (drug name) (amount) (unit of measurement of what's ordered) is ordered but I don't know (X) how many (units of measurement of what's on hand) that equals, but I do know (conversion factor).

Statement to figure out what is what for a dosage calculation: I know that (drug name) (amount) (unit of measurement / qualifier) is ordered but I don't know how it comes (X). But I do know or I have on hand (drug name) (amount) (unit of measurement / qualifier) comes in (amount / form)

Problem without a conversion example:

Ordered: Happypill 200 mg, PO, QD
On hand: Happypill 400 mg tablets

Using the math scaffold: a calculation is needed and the answer is going to be "anything else". No conversion is needed because I only have two different qualifiers, mg and tablets.

Using the statement to fill in the structure:

$$\frac{200\,mg}{X\,tab} = \frac{400\,mg}{1\,tab}$$

I know that Happypill 200 mg is ordered but I don't know how it comes (X). But I do know Happypill 400 mg comes in one tablet.

IMPORTANT: Notice that mg is on the top position on both sides. This is very important. The qualifier on the top on each side must match and the qualifier on the bottom on each side must match for this to work.

$$\frac{200\,mg}{X\,tab} \diagdown\!\!\!\!\!\diagup \frac{400\,mg}{1\,tab}$$

Now solve by cross-multiplying then solving for "X"

$$400x = 200$$

$$\frac{\cancel{400}}{\cancel{400}}x = \frac{2\cancel{00}}{4\cancel{00}}$$

Get "X" by itself by dividing both sides by 400

$$x = \frac{2}{4}$$

$$x = \frac{1}{2}\,tab$$

Reduce to get the final answer

Problem with a conversion example:

> Ordered: Happypill 0.2 g, PO, QD
> On hand: Happypill 400 mg tablets

Using the math scaffold: a calculation is needed and the answer is going to be "anything else". A conversion is needed because I have three different qualifiers g, mg, and tablets.

You can go ahead and draw two formula structures to remind you that there are going to be two calculations

Using the statement for a conversion:

$$\frac{0.2g}{X\,mg} = \frac{1g}{1000\,mg}$$

I know that Happypill 0.2 g is ordered but I don't know (X) how many mg that equals, but I do know that 1g equals 1000mg.

IMPORTANT: Notice that g is on the top on both sides. This is very important. The qualifier on the top on each side must match and the qualifier on the bottom on each side must match for this to work.

$$\frac{0.2g}{X\,mg} \times \frac{1g}{1000\,mg}$$

$$X = \frac{1000}{0.2}$$

$$\frac{}{200.0}$$

$$X = 200\,mg$$

Now solve by cross-multiplying then solving for "X". To be extra careful if you are calculating by hand you might want to do that calculation on the side to avoid decimal errors.

Now you know that 0.2 g = 200mg, the order is equivalent to Happypill 200mg. PO, QD

Using the math scaffold: a calculation is needed and the answer is going to be "anything else". No conversion is needed because I only have two different qualifiers, mg and tablets.

$$\frac{200\,mg}{X\,tab} = \frac{400\,mg}{1\,tab}$$

$$\frac{200\,mg}{X\,tab} \times \frac{400\,mg}{1\,tab}$$

$$400X = 200$$

$$\frac{400}{400}X = \frac{200}{400}$$

$$X = \frac{2}{4}$$

$$X = \frac{1}{2}\,tab$$

Using the statement to fill in the structure:
I know that Happypill 200 mg is ordered but I don't know how it comes (X). But I do know Happypill 400 mg comes in one tablet.

Now solve by cross-multiplying then solving for "X"

Get "X" by itself by dividing both sides by 400

Reduce to get the final answer

8 ✳ Desired over Have ✳ 8

The basic structure for Desired over Have is:

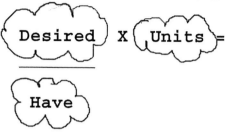

$$\frac{\text{Desired}}{\text{Have}} \times \text{Units} =$$

You start by identifying what is "Desired" that is what is ordered for the patient or specific to the patient in the question. You place the "desired" then the "have" is the other item with the same qualifier. The "Units" is related to the "Have". It is the partner of that component. Once everything is in its place you multiply across then divide to obtain your answer.

Problem without a conversion example:

Ordered: Happypill 200 mg, PO, QD
On hand: Happypill 400 mg tablets

Using the math scaffold: a calculation is needed and the answer is going to be "anything else". No conversion is needed because I only have two different qualifiers, mg and tablets.

$$\frac{200\,mg}{400\,mg} \times 1\,tab =$$

I *desire* 200 mg
I *have* 400 mg in 1 tablet (*units*)

IMPORTANT: Notice that mg is on the top and bottom in the first section of the problem. This is very important. The qualifier then cancels out and you are left with the qualifier in the second section. This will be the form your answer will be in. This is an important check that assures you have everything in the right place.

$$\frac{2\cancel{00}\,\cancel{mg}}{4\cancel{00}\,\cancel{mg}} \times 1\,tab = \frac{2}{4}\,tab$$

Now solve by multiplying across

$$\frac{2}{4}\,tab = \frac{1}{2}\,tab$$

Divide or Reduce to get the final answer

22

Problem with a conversion example:

Ordered: Happypill 0.2 g, PO, QD
On hand: Happypill 400 mg tablets

Using the math scaffold: a calculation is needed and the answer is going to be "anything else". A conversion is needed because I have three different qualifiers g, mg, and tablets.

You can go ahead and draw two formula structures to remind you that there are going to be two calculations

$$\frac{0.2g}{1g} \times 1000mg =$$

I *desire* 0.2g (Okay so you don't really desire it but it is what is specific to the patient)
I *have/know* 1g equals 1000mg (*units*)

IMPORTANT: Notice that g is on the top and bottom in the first section of the problem. This is very important. The qualifier then cancels out and you are left with the qualifier in the second section. This will be the form your answer will be in. This is an important check that assures you have everything in the right place.

$$\frac{0.2g}{1g} \times 1000mg = 0.2 \times 1000$$

Now solve by multiplying across

Divide or Reduce to get the conversion

$$\frac{1000}{0.2} = 200mg$$
$$200.0$$

Now you know that 0.2 g = 200mg, the order is equivalent to Happypill 200mg. PO, QD

Using the math scaffold: a calculation is needed and the answer is going to be "anything else". No conversion is needed because I only have two different qualifiers, mg and tablets.

$$\frac{200mg}{400mg} \times 1 tab =$$

I *desire* 200 mg
I *have* 400 mg in 1 tablet (*units*)

$$\frac{200 mg}{400 mg} \times 1 tab = \frac{2}{4} tab$$

Now solve by multiplying across

Divide or Reduce to get the final answer

$$\frac{2}{4} tab = \frac{1}{2} tab$$

23

9 ✳Dimensional Analysis ✳ 9

Dimensional Analysis basic structure is:

Dimensional Analysis starts with what is ordered or specific to the patient all by itself. The next section is for a conversion factor if necessary. The final section is for what is on hand. You look to the qualifiers to help you fill in the blanks. You can cancel out a qualifier if there is one on the top and one on the bottom. This also serves as a check that everything is placed correctly because once you have cancelled out the qualifiers the one left should be what your answer will be in. When the information is filled in and the qualifiers cancelled out you multiply across and then divide or reduce to get your answer. If no conversion is needed there will be only be two columns of numbers where as with a conversion there will be three.

Problem without a conversion example:

Ordered: Happypill 200 mg, PO, QD
On hand: Happypill 400 mg tablets

Using the math scaffold: a calculation is needed and the answer is going to be "anything else". No conversion is needed because I only have two different qualifiers, mg and tablets so only two columns are needed.

$$200mg \times \frac{}{mg}$$

Start with what is ordered

$$200mg \times \frac{1\ tab}{400mg}$$

The part of the "on hand" that is in mg must go on the bottom so I can cancel out mg. 400 goes with mg so I fill that number in. The partner to 400 mg is 1 tablet so that has to go on top of the 400 mg

$$200\ mg \times \frac{1\ tab}{400mg} = \frac{200}{400}\ tab$$

Now cancel out the qualifiers. I only have tablet left so that is the qualifier for my answer. Solve by multiplying across.

$$\frac{200}{400} = \frac{1}{2}\ tab$$

Divide or Reduce to get the final answer

Problem with a conversion example:

Ordered: Happypill 0.2 g, PO, QD
On hand: Happypill 400 mg tablets

Using the math scaffold: a calculation is needed and the answer is going to be "anything else". A conversion is needed because I have three different qualifiers g, mg, and tablets so in this case there will be three columns needed.

$$0.2g \times \frac{}{g} \times \frac{}{} =$$

Start with what is ordered. Because a conversion is needed from g to mg the next section is going to be the conversion factor.

$$0.2g \times \frac{1000\ mg}{1\ g} \times \frac{}{mg} =$$

$$0.2g \times \frac{1000\ mg}{1g} \times \frac{1\ tab}{400\ mg} =$$

Because I want to cancel out g I know 1 g goes on the bottom. The partner in the conversion factor goes on the top, in this case 1000 mg. The part of the "on hand" that is in mg must go on the bottom so I can cancel out mg. 400 goes with mg so I fill in that number. The partner to 400 mg is 1 tablet so that has to go on top of the 400 mg

$$0.2\cancel{g} \times \frac{1000\ \cancel{mg}}{1\cancel{g}} \times \frac{1\ tab}{400\ \cancel{mg}} = \frac{200\ tab}{400}$$

Now cancel out the qualifiers. I only have tablet left so that is the qualifier for my answer. Solve by multiplying across.

$$\frac{200}{400}\ tab = \frac{1}{2}\ tab$$

Reduce / divide to get the final answer

10 ✳ Practice with the Fab Four ✳ 10

Now that all four methods have been explained its time to work through ten basic calculation problems using the math scaffold and all four methods. Remember, this is a very important step so approach it with and open mind and more importantly do it! More complex problems dealing with reconstitution, meds based on weight, mixing meds, and the all important IV medication drip questions are found in the next chapter.

Practice all Four Question One

Ordered: Namenda 20 mg, PO, QD
On hand: Namenda 10 mg tablets

Solve using Ratio-Proportion	Solve using Fraction Method

Ordered: Namenda 20 mg, PO, QD
On hand: Namenda 10 mg tablets

Solve using Desired over Have	Solve using Dimensional Analysis

Practice all Four Question Two

Ordered: Morphine 4 mg, IV, Q4H prn pain
On hand: Morphine 10 mg /ml

Solve using Ratio-Proportion	Solve using Fraction Method

Ordered: Morphine 4 mg, IV, Q4H prn pain
On hand: Morphine 10 mg /ml

Solve using Desired over Have	Solve using Dimensional Analysis

Practice all Four Question Three

Ordered: Potassium Chloride oral solution 20 mEq, PO, BID
On hand: Potassium Chloride oral solution 40 mEq / 15 ml

Solve using Ratio-Proportion	Solve using Fraction Method

Ordered: Potassium Chloride oral solution 20 mEq, PO, BID
On hand: Potassium Chloride oral solution 40 mEq / 15 ml

Solve using Desired over Have	Solve using Dimensional Analysis

Practice all Four Question Four

Ordered: Lasix 40 mg, IV, QD
On hand: Lasix 10 mg / ml

Solve using Ratio-Proportion	Solve using Fraction Method

Ordered: Lasix 40 mg, IV, QD
On hand: Lasix 10 mg / ml

Solve using Desired over Have	Solve using Dimensional Analysis

Practice all Four Question Five

Ordered: Hydrochlorathyazide 12.5 mg, PO, BID
On hand: Hydrochlorathyazide 25 mg tablets

Solve using Ratio-Proportion	Solve using Fraction Method

Ordered: Hydrochlorathyazide 12.5 mg, PO, BID
On hand: Hydrochlorathyazide 25 mg tablets

Solve using Desired over Have	Solve using Dimensional Analysis

Practice all Four Question Six

Ordered: Digoxin 0.125 mg, PO, QD
On hand: Digoxin 0.25 mg tablets

Solve using Ratio-Proportion	Solve using Fraction Method

Ordered: Digoxin 0.125 mg, PO, QD
On hand: Digoxin 0.25 mg tablets

Solve using Desired over Have	Solve using Dimensional Analysis

Practice all Four Question Seven

Ordered: Synthroid 50 mcg, PO, QD
On hand: Synthroid 0.025 mg tablets

Solve using Ratio-Proportion	Solve using Fraction Method

Ordered: Synthroid 50 mcg, PO, QD
On hand: Synthroid 0.025 mg tablets

Solve using Desired over Have	Solve using Dimensional Analysis

Practice all Four Question Eight

Ordered: Atropine gr 1/150 , IM, on call to OR
On hand: Atropine 0.4 mg / ml

Solve using Ratio-Proportion	Solve using Fraction Method

Ordered: Atropine gr 1/150 , IM, on call to OR
On hand: Atropine 0.4 mg / ml

Solve using Desired over Have	Solve using Dimensional Analysis

Practice all Four Question Nine

Ordered: Acetazolamide 1gm, PO, Now
On hand: Acetazolamide 500 mg tablets

Solve using Ratio-Proportion	Solve using Fraction Method

Ordered: Acetazolamide 1gm, PO, Now
On hand: Acetazolamide 500 mg tablets

Solve using Desired over Have	Solve using Dimensional Analysis

Practice all Four Question Ten

Ordered: Heparin 5000 units, SQ, Q12h
On hand: Heparin 10,000 units / ml

Solve using Ratio-Proportion	Solve using Fraction Method

Ordered: Heparin 5000 units, SQ, Q12h
On hand: Heparin 10,000 units / ml

Solve using Desired over Have	Solve using Dimensional Analysis

Quick Answers

These are the quick answers. To see the problems all worked out all four ways go to the answer section in the back of the book.

1. 2 tablets
2. 0.4 ml
3. 7.5 ml
4. 4 ml
5. 0.5 tablets
6. 0.5 tablets
7. 2 tablets
8. 1 ml
9. 2 tablets
10. 0.5 ml

11 ✴ More Complex Anything Else Problems ✴ 11

These problems tend to confuse students because they are typically a longer narrative, have information that you don't need to do the math, and aren't usually set up in the ordered / on-hand way. This is because the questions generally mimic how real life clinical situations are presented to you. These are questions you will see a lot of especially the IV medication questions. Since your answer will be something other than gtts/min all of these questions will be solved with your anything else formula.

Reconstitution Questions

Reconstitution is simply putting the medication back into solution from a powder form. Some medications are unstable in solution for long periods and this extends their shelf life. So you just mix it when you need it and use it right away. Much like mixing koolaid you start with powder, have to follow the directions to mix it to the right concentration. With medications you may even have a choice of concentrations. The vial containing the powder will have instructions usually in a grid if there is a choice of concentrations to achieve. You then choose which one works best for your situation. The vial will also usually have the total amount of medication in the vial listed.

Ordered: AntibioticX 250 mg, IM now
On Hand: AntibioticX 1g / vial in a dry powder. Instructions for reconstitution read: add sterile normal saline as follows to achieve the appropriate concentration.

Concentration	Diluent	Total volume
200 mg/ml	4.7	5 ml
500mg/ml	1.7 ml	2 ml

Okay, as you can see there are more numbers to choose from and its starting to look scary. All the grid is saying is if you add 4.7 ml of fluid you will end up with 5 ml of medication that will have 200 mg / ml and if you add 1.7 ml you will end up with 2 ml of medication that will have 500mg / ml. Let's look at what you have here in terms of what information you don't need and what you do need.

What you don't need:
1. The total amount in the whole vial (1g) it will not be in your calculation
2. The amount of diluent to add (4.7 or 1.7) it will not be part of your calculation. In real life you will be drawing up one of those amounts and injecting it into the vial. On a test you just pretend you have reconstituted the medication and look to the final concentration outcome.
3. The total volume (5 ml or 2 ml) it will not be part of your calculation

What you do need:
1. The concentration you decide to use based on the patient situation or making the math easier. In most cases the patient would much rather receive a smaller amount IM than a larger amount. And if you reconstitute it to a volume greater than allowed to give in one injection it will mean two injections for the patient. In this case neither concentrations

will pose a problem with the volumes for the dose that is ordered but since 500 is divisible by 250 lets choose that concentration to make the math easy.

All you need to look at in all of that information is the ordered amount and the concentration you chose.

Ordered: AntibioticX 250 mg, IM Now
On hand: AntibioticX 500 mg /ml

Try finding the answer now with your anything else formula. Look for the answer worked out in all four ways in the answer section in the back of the book

Questions Using Weight to Determine Dosage

Some medications are given based on the patient's weight. This is frequently the case with children. This is a two step process

1. The first step is to obtain the patient's weight in kilograms (kg) and translate the order for that person's weight
2. Now calculate the what you will give the patient based on what you have on hand

Ordered: Ibuprofen 10 mg /kg, Q6H, prn temp >102, child weighs 44 lbs
On hand: Ibuprofen 100 mg / 5 ml

First step is to find the dose of ibuprofen for a child that weighs 44 lbs by converting the weight to kg using your anything else formula. The order of 10 mg / kg simply means for each kg of body weight give 10 mg of the medicine. You can find the weight in kg using your anything else formula and multiply by 10 to get the amount ordered for the patient. If you want you can use your anything else formula again to find the amount. Finally you will use your anything else formula one more time to find how many ml you will administer.

If you use Dimensional Analysis it is like an all inclusive vacation, everything is included in one formula, converting the weight, calculating the dosage, and what you will be giving the patient all in one.

Try finding the answer now with your anything else formula. Look for the answer worked out in all four ways in the answer section in the back of the book

Mixing Medications Questions

To save giving the patient two injections sometimes medications are mixed into the same syringe. It is okay to do this as long as the medications are compatible with each other and the total volume does not exceed volume limits of injections. So this is not a difficult kind of problem it simply will require two separate calculations to find out how much of each medication you will be given. It may ask you to add the total volumes at the end, nothing fancy needed to do that.

Ordered: Meperidine 20 mg and Promethazine 10, IM, On call to the OR
On hand: Meperidine 50 mg / ml and Promethazine 25 mg / ml

Try finding the answer now with your anything else formula. Look for the answer worked out in all four ways in the answer section in the back of the book

You will give ____ml of Meperidine and ____ml of Promethezine for a total injection volume of ____ml

Questions Involving Continuous IV Medication Infusions

You will definitely run into these questions on calculation tests and in clinical. Don't get nervous that the medication is in an IV bag. Follow the math scaffold and you will know what to do. If the answer is going to be units/hr, ml/hr, mg/hr....anything but gtts/min what do you use? Your anything else formula!! Students tend to see "IV" and automatically go to the IV formula. Just because it involves an IV bag does not mean it will be a gtts/min answer. Read the question all the way through and determine if the answer will be gtts/min or anything else. Another thing that makes these confusing is that often teachers will show you a different approach to calculating these problems involving either multiplying or dividing by the concentration factor. Why learn and try to remember two ways of doing something that you can accomplish using your anything else formula? Keep using your anything else formula!

Another thing to keep in mind with these questions is that they don't necessarily have what is ordered or specific to the patient positioned in the first part of the question, it may come towards the end. So remember to look for what is ordered or specific to the patient not just the first number that comes along. The "something" per hour is usually the ordered or specific to the patient number.

Examples of this phenomenon:

Question One:
A patient has a continuous heparin infusion. The bag is labeled Heparin 25,000 units in 500ml NS and is infusing at **24 ml/hr**. How many units per hour of Heparin is the patient receiving?

OR

A patient has a continuous heparin infusion running at **24 ml/hr**. The bag is labeled Heparin 25,000 units in 500ml NS. How many units per hour of Heparin is the patient receiving?

Question Two:
The patient is to receive Heparin **1000 units/hr**. The bag is labeled Heparin 25,000 units in 250 ml of NS. How many ml/hr should the patient receive?

OR

The patient has a bag labeled Heparin 25,000 units in 250ml NS hanging. What should the IV pump be set at to deliver **1000 units/hr**? (this version even brings in an IV pump. All continuous medication infusions should be given via an IV pump and all pumps are set by ml/hr)

A note about qualifiers: Usually we only want 2 different qualifiers or we know a conversion is needed. In these kinds of problems think of time as the third dimension rather than the third qualifier. In basic problems you only want to be left with one qualifier at the end. In these questions you keep the time qualifier because it is in your answer.

51

Examples of solving Questions 1 & 2 using all four formulas

Question 1

Ratio-Proportion

$24 \text{ ml/hr} : X \text{ units} = 500 \text{ ml} : 25,000 \text{ units}$

$24 \text{ ml/hr} : X \text{ units} = 500 \text{ ml} : 25,000 \text{ units}$

$$500 X = \begin{array}{r} 25,000 \\ \times 24 \\ \hline 100000 \\ 50000 \\ \hline 600000 \end{array}$$

$$\frac{\cancel{500}}{\cancel{500}} X = \frac{600000}{\cancel{500}}$$

$$X = 5\overline{)6000} \quad \begin{array}{r} 1200 \\ \underline{5} \\ 10 \\ \underline{10} \\ 0 \end{array} \qquad X = 1200 \text{ units/hr}$$

I know 24 ml is ordered but I don't know how many units that is but I do know that 500 ml has 25,000 units

Multiply means and extremes

Be careful with big numbers. Do calculations on the side as I did if you aren't using a calculator

Reduce / divide to get your answer

Fraction Method

$$\frac{24 \text{ ml/hr}}{X \text{ units}} = \frac{500 \text{ ml}}{25,000 \text{ units}}$$

$$\frac{24 \text{ ml/hr}}{X \text{ units}} \times \frac{500 \text{ ml}}{25,000 \text{ units}}$$

$$5 X = \begin{array}{r} 250 \\ \times 24 \\ \hline 1000 \\ 500 \\ \hline 6000 \end{array}$$

$$\frac{\cancel{5}}{\cancel{5}} x = \frac{6000}{5} = 5\overline{)6000} \begin{array}{r} 1200 \\ \underline{5} \\ 10 \\ \underline{10} \\ 0 \end{array}$$

$$X = 1200 \text{ units/hr}$$

I know 24 ml is ordered but I don't know how many units that is but I do know that 500 ml has 25,000 units

Cross multiply

Be careful with big numbers. Do calculations on the side as I did if you aren't using a calculator

Reduce / divide to get your answer

Desired over Have

$$\frac{24 \text{ ml/hr}}{500 \text{ ml}} \times 25000 \text{ units} =$$

$$\frac{24 \text{ ml/hr}}{500 \text{ ml}} \times 25000 \text{ units} = \frac{600,000}{500} \text{ units/hr}$$

$$= 5\overline{)6000} \begin{array}{r} 1200 \\ \underline{5} \\ 10 \\ \underline{10} \\ 0 \end{array} = 1200 \text{ units/hr}$$

24 ml is desired, I have 500 ml with 25,000 units

Multiply across

Be careful with big numbers. Do calculations on the side as I did if you aren't using a calculator

Reduce / divide to get your answer

Dimensional Analysis

$$24 \, ml/hr \times \frac{\quad\quad}{ml} =$$

$$24 \, ml/hr \times \frac{25000 \, units}{500 \, ml} = \frac{6000}{5} \, units/hr$$

$$5\overline{)6000} \quad\begin{array}{c}1200\end{array} = 1200 \, units/hr$$
$$\begin{array}{c}5\\\overline{10}\\10\\\overline{0}\end{array}$$

24 ml is ordered . I know now that 500 ml will go on the bottom so ml will cancel out. The partner of 500 ml is 25,000 units so that goes on top

Multiply across

Be careful with big numbers. Do calculations on the side as I did if you aren't using a calculator

Reduce / divide to get your answer

Question 2

Ratio-Proportion

$$1000 \, units/hr : X \, ml = 25000 \, units : 250 \, ml$$

$$1000 \, units/hr : X \, ml = 25000 \, units : 250 \, ml$$

$$25000 \, X = 250,000$$

$$\frac{25000}{25000} X = \frac{250000}{25000}$$

$$= 10 \, ml/hr$$

I know 1000units is ordered but I don't know how many ml that is but I do know that 25000 units is in 250 ml

Multiply means and extremes

Be careful with big numbers. Do calculations on the side as I did if you aren't using a calculator

Reduce / divide to get your answer

Fraction Method

$$\frac{1000 \, units/hr}{X \, ml} = \frac{25000 \, units}{250 \, ml}$$

$$\frac{1000 \, units/hr}{X \, ml} \times \frac{25000 \, units}{250 \, ml}$$

$$25,000 \, X = 250,000$$

$$\frac{25,000}{25000} X = \frac{250000}{25000}$$

$$X = 10 \, ml/hr$$

I know 1000 unitsis ordered but I don't know how many ml that is but I do know that 25,000 units is in 250 ml

Cross multiply

Be careful with big numbers. Do calculations on the side as I did if you aren't using a calculator

Reduce / divide to get your answer

Desired over Have

$$\frac{1000 \, units/hr}{25000 \, units} \times 250 \, ml =$$

$$\frac{1000 \, units/hr}{25000 \, units} \times 250 \, ml = \frac{250}{25}$$

$$= 10 \, ml/hr$$

1000 units is desired, I have 25,000units in 250 ml

Multiply across

Be careful with big numbers. Do calculations on the side as I did if you aren't using a calculator

Reduce / divide to get your answer

53

Dimensional Analysis

$$1000 \text{ units/hr} \times \underline{\hspace{2cm}} = $$
$$\qquad\qquad\qquad \text{units}$$

$$1000 \text{ units/hr} \times \frac{250 \text{ ml}}{25000 \text{ units}} = \frac{250000}{25000}$$

$$= 10 \text{ ml/hr}$$

1000 units are ordered . I know now that 25,000 units will go on the bottom so units will cancel out. The partner of 25,000 units is 250 ml so that goes on top

Multiply across

Be careful with big numbers. Do calculations on the side as I did if you aren't using a calculator

Reduce / divide to get your answer

Quick!! Try a few Medication Infusion Questions using your "anything else" formula. Keep in mind there are many ways for instructors to configure these questions.

1. Order: Infuse Heparin at 1400 units per hour, Bag on hand 25,000 units in 250 ml NS.

2. Patient has an aminophylline drip labeled 500 mg in 250 ml NS running at 15 ml / hr. How much aminophylline is the patient receiving per hour?

3. The patient has a continuous Heparin infusion labeled Heparin 25,000 units in NS 500 ml How many units per is the patient receiving if the infusion is running at 16 ml per hour?

12 ✱ Classic IV Formula ✱ 12

We have spent a lot of time and gone through a lot of problems focusing on "Anything Else" answers. Now it is time to look at what to do if your answer will be gtts/min. Sometimes this is referred to as the flow rate or gtts/min may be written out as drops per minute.

Here's the classic IV formula:

$$\frac{\text{Total Volume in ml}}{\text{Total Time in Min.}} \quad \text{X} \quad \text{GTT Factor}$$

The three items you need are total volume of the infusion in **milliliters,** the total time in **minutes** and the **drop factor.** Once these are identified you simply multiply across then divide to find your answer. How you find these items in questions and in clinical may be a bit different. Let's look at the three items individually.

Milliliters—Real orders for IV's are frequently written as ml / hr so that is your volume. The other situation is an intermittent infusion or piggyback. In that case the pharmacy rather than the physician generally determines how much fluid to put the drug in for the infusion so look on the bag itself for the volume. Occasionally you might be given an order for a bolus of fluid such as 500ml over two hours. In that case the 500ml is your total volume in ml. For exams often you will be given odd things like infuse 1 L over 12 hours or 1.5 liters in 24 hours. In these situations you will need to convert the liters to milliliters by multiplying by 1000. Fluid names much like drug names don't play a part in the calculation but because they are unfamiliar to you and some contain numbers they can cause confusion. Common IV fluids abbreviations and what they mean are:

Abbreviation	Interpretation
D5W	Dextrose 5% in Water
D5 ½ NS	Dextrose 5% in 0.45% Saline solution
D5NS	Dextrose 5% in 0.9% Saline solution
NS	0.9% Saline solution
½ NS	0.45% Saline solution
LR	Lactated Ringers solution
D5LR	Dextrose 5% in Lactated Ringers solution

Also, sometimes the total volume of the bag is in the question as well as the ml / hr. In that case you can ignore the total volume of the bag because it is just extra information when you have the ml / hr.

Minutes—If it is ordered as ml / hr that is the volume specified to infuse over 60 minutes on a continuous basis so your time is 60 minutes. If it is an intermittent infusion again the pharmacy or a drug reference will give you the infusion time (such as infuse over 30 minutes) rather than the physician order. On a test that information will be given to you, in clinical you will have to look at the bag, consult your drug guide or the pharmacist.

Drop Factor—What is a drop factor in the first place? IV tubing has what is called a drip chamber at the top where it plugs into the bag of fluid. The size of the opening at the top of the drip chamber determines the size of the drops. The drop factor is the number of drops it takes to equal one milliliter. Minidrip tubing is 60 gtts/ml. Maxidrip tubing can be 10, 15, or 20 gtts/ml. In clinical this information is found on the tubing package or for tubing already hanging. Usually a facility only uses one size for maxidrop so if you look in the supply room for a package of tubing with the same drip chamber you will be able to determine this information. On a test they must give you this information. The IV tubing is also called the infusion "set". It's the set of equipment used to infuse the fluids.

IV tubing drip chambers

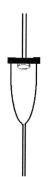

You can tell a maxidrop tubing set by the large opening from which drops fall. However, maxidrop tubing can be 10, 15, or 20 gtts per ml. The larger the drop the fewer drops it takes to make 1 ml.

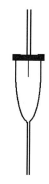

You can tell a minidrop tubing set by the needle like projection from which drops fall. Minidrip tubing is always 60 gtts / ml. The drops are much smaller and it takes 60 gtts to make 1 ml.

Frequently you will have IV pumps to work with. IV pumps are machines that you thread the tubing into and it pumps the fluid at a rate you program it to deliver. IV pumps are programmed to deliver milliliters per hour. Some pumps can even be set to one decimal point. This is used when you are infusing small amounts of very potent medications or for babies. So you might see a pump set for 7.5 ml / hr for example. While pumps are widely used you will still have to run some items "by gravity". That's what it called when you calculate the drops/ minute and regulate the flow by using the roller clamp. For example if you calculated your drops per minute (gtts/min) to be 16 you will open the roller clamp while watching the drops fall in the drop chamber. Using your watch you will count the drops and manipulate the roller clamp until you have 16 drops falling per minute. This skill takes some practice. While it has nothing to do with the math part I strongly recommend you practice regulating an IV by gravity in your nursing lab. Any equipment or procedures you are comfortable with prior to doing at a real patient's bedside will make your clinical experience much less stressful and more productive.

Back to Math! Here are some examples of IV flow rate questions.

1. Calculate the flow rate (gtts/min) to infuse D5W at 124 ml/hr, using a 10 gtt / ml set

Using the math scaffold: a calculation is needed and the answer is going to be "gtts / min" so we use the classic IV formula

Milliliters = 124
Minutes = 60
Drop Factor= 10

$$\frac{124}{60} \times 10 = \frac{1240}{60}$$

$$60\overline{)1240} \quad \begin{array}{r} 20.6 \\ \underline{120} \\ 40 \\ \underline{0} \\ 400 \\ \underline{360} \\ 40 \end{array} \quad = 21 \text{ gtts/min}$$

2. NS 1000 ml to infuse at 40 ml / hr using a microdrip

Using the math scaffold: a calculation is needed and the answer is going to be "gtts / min" so we use the classic IV formula

Milliliters = 40
Minutes = 60
Drop Factor = 60

$$\frac{40}{60} \times 60 =$$

Something multiplied by 60 then divided by 60 is the original number so a nice thing about 60 gtt sets is the ml per hour = gtts per minute

$$\frac{40}{60} \times 60 = 40 \text{ gtts/min}$$

3. Lactated Ringer's 500 ml infuse over 2 hours using a 10 gtt set

Using the math scaffold: a calculation is needed and the answer is going to be "gtts / min" so we use the classic IV formula

Milliliters = 500
Minutes = 120
Drop Factor = 10

$$\frac{500}{120} \times 10 =$$

$$\frac{500}{120} \times 10 = \frac{500}{12}$$

$$\begin{array}{r} 41.6 \\ 12\overline{)500} \\ \underline{48} \\ 20 \\ \underline{12} \\ 80 \\ \underline{72} \\ 80 \end{array} = 42 \text{ gtts/min}$$

In this situation you must remember to change the hours to minutes

4. Ancef 1 gram IVPB. You have a bag labeled Ancef 1 g in 50 ml NS infuse over 30 minutes using a 10 gtt set.

Using the math scaffold: a calculation is needed and the answer is going to be "gtts / min" so we use the classic IV formula

Milliliters = 50
Minutes = 30
Drop Factor = 10

$$\frac{50}{30} \times 10 =$$

$$\frac{50}{30} \times 10 = \frac{50}{3}$$

$$\begin{array}{r} 16.6 \\ 3\overline{)50} \\ \underline{3} \\ 20 \\ \underline{18} \\ 20 \\ \underline{18} \\ 2 \end{array} = 17 \text{ gtts/min}$$

This situation has extra information not relevant to your calculation. Don't let that confuse you.

57

5. D5LR with 1 amp MVI infuse at 125 ml / hour using a 15 gtt set.

Using the math scaffold: a calculation is needed and the answer is going to be "gtts / min" so we use the classic IV formula

Milliliters = 125
Minutes = 60
Drop Factor = 15

$$\frac{125}{60} \times 15 = \frac{1875}{60} = 60\overline{\smash)1875.}\,^{31.25} = 31\ gtts/min$$

$$\begin{array}{r} 31.25 \\ 60\overline{\smash)1875.} \\ \underline{180} \\ 75 \\ \underline{68} \\ 150 \\ \underline{120} \\ 300 \end{array}$$

Again additional information may confuse you. The 1 amp MVI is simply an amount of Multivitamin added to the IV bag and isn't a part of your calculation.

13 ✳ Additional Practice Questions A-Z ✳ 13

A. Ordered: Aprazolam 0.5 mg, PO, TID, PRN
   On Hand: Aprazolam 1 mg tablets

B. Ordered: Bumex 1 mg IVP daily
   On hand: Bumex 0.25 mg / ml

C. Ordered: Carbamazepine 150 mg PO BID
   On Hand:Carbamazepine 100 mg / 5 ml oral suspension

D. Digoxin 0.25 mg IV daily
   0.5 mg / 2 ml

E. Erythromycin 500 mg PO Q12H
   Erythromycin 250 mg tablets

F. Furosemide 30 mg PO daily
   Furosemide 20 mg tablets

G. Guanfacine 2mg PO Daily
   Guanfacine 1 mg tablets

H. Ordered: Heparin 5000 units IVP now then start Heparin infusion at 800 units per hour
   On Hand: Vial labeled heparin 1000 units per ml and bag labeled 25,000 units Heparin in 250 ml
   NS (Hint: you have two things here what you will draw up in the syringe for the bolus and what
   you will set the IV pump at to deliver the dose)

I. Ordered: Ibuprofen 600 mg PO Q6H PRN
   On Hand: Ibuprofen 200 mg tablets

J. Jog, jump, walk a journey, play on a jungle gym, just do it! Keeping physically fit will help
   prevent injury and give you the stamina to make it through a 12 hour shift. (Can you believe
   how unpopular the letter J is when it comes to drug names?)

K. Ordered: Ketoconazole 400 mg PO daily
   On Hand: Ketoconazole 200 mg tablets

L. Ordered: Lactulose 30 grams PO TID
   On Hand: Lactulose 10 grams / 15 ml

M. Ordered: Methylprednisolone 40 mg
   On Hand: Methylprednisolone 125 mg / ml

N. Ordered: Naloxone 0.1 mg IV STAT
   On Hand: Naloxone 0.4 mg / ml

O. Ordered: Omeprazole 40 mg PO Daily
   On Hand: Omprazole 20 mg tablets

P. Ordered: Penicillin G 1,000,000 units Q4H IVPB
   On Hand: Bag labeled Penicillin G 1,000,000 units in 50 ml NS infuse over 20 minutes and microdrip IV tubing (60 gtt = 1 ml) Calculate the gtts/min

Q. Ordered: Quinidine 250 mg Q6H
   On Hand: Quinidine 100 mg tablets

R. Ordered: Rifampin 600 mg PO Daily
   On Hand: Rifampin 300 mg tablets

S. Ordered: Sucralfate 500 mg PO TID AC
   On Hand: Sucralfate 1 gram tablets

T. Ordered: Ticarcillin / Clavulanate 3 g /100 mg IVPB Q4H
   On Hand: Bag labeled Ticarcillin / Clavulante 3 g / 100 mg in 50 ml NS infuse over 30 minutes and 10 gtt/ml IV set. Calculate the gtts/min

U. "U" can't text me but "U" can email me at Karen@nursethings.com if you need the worked out version of the answer for any of the practice problems

V. Ordered: Verapamil 100 mcg / kg IV Now
   On Hand: Verapamil 2.5 mg / ml, patient weighs 198 lbs

W. Ordered: Warfarin 7.5 mg PO Today
   On Hand: Warfarin 5 mg tablets

X. Xylophone is a musical instrument. Maintain some interests like playing a musical instrument while in nursing school.

Y. You can do it!

Z. Ordered: Zidovudine 300 mg PO BID
   On Hand: Zidovudine 100 mg capsules

14 ✻ A Few Grain Questions Just in Case ✻ 14

1. Ordered Codeine gr ½ Q4H prn, pain
   On hand: Codeine 15 mg tablets

2. Ordered Phenobarbital liquid gr 1/6 PO TID
   On Hand: Phenobarbital liquid 20 mg / 5ml

3. Ordered: Scopolamine gr 1/100 PO Q12H
   On hand: Scopolamine 0.6 mg Tablets

4. Ordered: Phenobarbital gr ¾ PO QID
   On Hand: Phenobarbital 30 mg tablets

15 ✻ Extra IV Flowrate Questions ✻ 15

Calculate the gtts/min to deliver the following IV infusions. Calculate each one for the four different IV sets.

IV Order	Using 10gtts/ml set	Using 15gtts/ml set	Using 20gtts/ml set	Using 60gtts/ml set
D5NS at 100 ml /hr				
NS at 125 ml / hr				
LR at 50 ml / hr				
½ NS 500 ml to infuse over 3 hrs				

16 ✳ Answer Section ✳ 16

Answers to Practice Questions A-Z

A) ½ tablet

B) 4 ml

C) 7.5 ml

D) 1 ml

E) 2 tablets

F) 1.5 tablets

G) 2 tablets

H) 5 ml bolus, 8 ml / hr

I) 3 tablets

K) 2 tablets

L) 45 ml

M) 0.32 ml

N) 0.25 ml

O) 2 tablets

P) 150 gtts /min

Q) 2.5 tablets

R) 2 tablets

S) ½ tablet

T) 17 gtts/ min

V) 3.6 ml

W) 1.5 tablets

Z) 3 capsules

Answers to Extra Grain Questions

1) 2 tabs   2) 2.5 ml   3) 1 tablet   4) 1.5 tablets

Answers to Extra IV Flowrate Questions

IV Order	Using 10gtts/ml set	Using 15gtts/ml set	Using 20gtts/ml set	Using 60gtts/ml set
D5NS at 100 ml /hr	17 gtts/min	25 gtts/min	33 gtts/min	100 gtts/min
NS at 125 ml / hr	21 gtts/min	31 gtts/min	42 gtts/min	125 gtts/min
LR at 50 ml / hr	8 gtts/min	13 gtts/min	17 gtts/min	50 gtts/min
½ NS 500 ml to infuse over 3 hrs	28 gtts/min	42 gtts/min	56 gtts/min	167 gtts/min

Practice all Four Question One Answer

Ordered: Namenda 20 mg, PO, QD
On hand: Namenda 10 mg tablets

Ratio-Proportion

$20 \, mg : X \, tab = 10 \, mg : 1 \, tab$

$20 \, mg : X \, tab = 10 \, mg : 1 \, tab$

$10 \, x = 20$

$\dfrac{10}{10} x = \dfrac{20}{10}$

$x = 2 \, tab$

Fraction Method

$\dfrac{20 \, mg}{X \, tab} = \dfrac{10 \, mg}{1 \, tab}$

$\dfrac{20 \, mg}{X \, tab} \diagdown\!\!\!\diagup \dfrac{10 \, mg}{1 \, tab}$

$10 \, x = 20$

$\dfrac{10}{10} x = \dfrac{20}{10}$

$x = 2 \, tabs$

Desired over Have

$\dfrac{20 \, mg}{10 \, mg} \times 1 \, tab =$

$\dfrac{20 \, mg}{10 \, mg} \times 1 \, tab = \dfrac{20}{10} \, tab$

$= 2 \, tabs$

Dimensional Analysis

$20 \, mg \times \dfrac{\quad}{mg} =$

$20 \, mg \times \dfrac{1 \, tab}{10 \, mg} = \dfrac{20}{10} \, tab$

$= 2 \, tab$

Practice all Four Question Two Answer

Ordered: Morphine 4 mg, IV, Q4H prn pain
On hand: Morphine 10 mg /ml

Ratio-Proportion

$$4 \, mg : X \, ml = 10 \, mg : 1 \, ml$$

$$4 \, mg : X \, ml = 10 \, mg : 1 \, ml$$

$$10 X = 4$$

$$\frac{10}{10} X = \frac{4}{10}$$

$$X = 0.4 \, ml$$

Fraction Method

$$\frac{4 \, mg}{X \, ml} = \frac{10 \, mg}{1 \, ml}$$

$$\frac{4 \, mg}{X \, ml} \diagdown \frac{10 \, mg}{1 \, ml}$$

$$10 x = 4$$

$$\frac{10}{10} X = \frac{4}{10}$$

$$x = 0.4 \, ml$$

Desired over Have

$$\frac{4 \, mg}{10 \, mg} \times 1 \, ml =$$

$$\frac{4 \, mg}{10 \, mg} \times 1 \, ml = \frac{4}{10} \, ml$$

$$= 0.4 \, ml$$

Dimensional Analysis

$$4 \, mg \times \frac{\quad}{mg} =$$

$$4 \, mg \times \frac{1 \, ml}{10 \, mg} = \frac{4}{10} \, ml$$

$$= 0.4 \, ml$$

Practice all Four Question Three Answer

Ordered: Potassium Chloride oral solution 20 mEq, PO, BID
On hand: Potassium Chloride oral solution 40 mEq / 15 ml

Ratio-Proportion

$20 mEq : X ml = 40 mEq : 15 ml$

$20 mEq : X ml = 40 mEq : 15 ml$

$40 X = 300$

$\dfrac{40}{40} X = \dfrac{300}{40}$

$X = 7.5 ml$

Fraction Method

$\dfrac{20 mEq}{X ml} = \dfrac{40 mEq}{15 ml}$

$\dfrac{20 mEq}{X ml} \times \dfrac{40 mEq}{15 ml}$

$40 X = 300$

$\dfrac{40}{40} X = \dfrac{300}{40}$

$X = 7.5 ml$

Desired over Have

$\dfrac{20 mEq}{40 mEq} \times 15 ml =$

$\dfrac{20 mEq}{40 mEq} \times 15 ml = \dfrac{300}{40} ml$

$= 7.5 ml$

Dimensional Analysis

$20 mEq \times \dfrac{}{mEq} =$

$20 mEq \times \dfrac{15 ml}{40 mEq} = \dfrac{300}{40} ml$

$= 7.5 ml$

Practice all Four Question Four Answer

Ordered: Lasix 40 mg, IV, QD
On hand: Lasix 10 mg / ml

Ratio-Proportion

$40mg : X ml = 10 mg : 1 ml$

$40 mg : X ml = 10 mg : 1 ml$

$10 X = 40$

$\dfrac{10}{10} X = \dfrac{40}{10}$

$X = 4 ml$

Fraction Method

$\dfrac{40mg}{X ml} = \dfrac{10mg}{1 ml}$

$\dfrac{40mg}{X ml} \diagup\!\!\!\!\diagdown \dfrac{10mg}{1 ml}$

$10 x = 40$

$\dfrac{10}{16} x = \dfrac{40}{10}$

$x = 4 ml$

Desired over Have

$\dfrac{40mg}{10 mg} \times 1 ml =$

$\dfrac{40mg}{10mg} \times 1 ml = \dfrac{40}{10} ml$

$= 4 ml$

Dimensional Analysis

$40 mg \times \dfrac{}{mg} =$

$40 mg \times \dfrac{1 ml}{10 mg} = \dfrac{40}{10} ml$

$= 4 ml$

66

Practice all Four Question Five Answer

Ordered: Hydrochlorathyazide 12.5 mg, PO, BID
On hand: Hydrochlorathyazide 25 mg tablets

Ratio-Proportion

12.5mg : X tab = 25mg : 1 tab

12.5mg : X tab = 25mg : 1 tab

$$25X = 12.5$$

$$\frac{25}{25}X = \frac{12.5}{25} \qquad 25\overline{\smash{)}12.5} \quad \overset{.5}{}$$
$$\frac{12\ 5}{0}$$

$$X = 0.5 \text{ tab}$$

Fraction Method

$$\frac{12.5mg}{X \text{ tab}} = \frac{25mg}{1 \text{ tab}}$$

$$\frac{12.5mg}{X \text{ tab}} \times \frac{25mg}{1 \text{ tab}}$$

$$25X = 12.5$$

$$\frac{25}{25}X = \frac{12.5}{25} \qquad 25\overline{\smash{)}12.5} \quad \overset{.5}{}$$
$$\frac{12\ 5}{0}$$

$$X = 0.5 \text{ tab}$$

Desired over Have

$$\frac{12.5mg}{25 mg} \times 1 \text{ tab} =$$

$$\frac{12.5 mg}{25 mg} \times 1 \text{ tab} = \frac{12.5}{25} \text{ tab}$$

$$25\overline{\smash{)}12.5} \quad \overset{.5}{} = 0.5 \text{ tab}$$
$$\frac{12\ 5}{0}$$

Dimensional Analysis

$$12.5mg \times \frac{\quad}{mg} =$$

$$12.5mg \times \frac{1 \text{ tab}}{25 mg} = \frac{12.5}{25}$$

$$25\overline{\smash{)}12.5} \quad \overset{.5}{} = 0.5 \text{ tab}$$
$$\frac{12\ 5}{0}$$

67

Practice all Four Question Six Answer

Ordered: Digoxin 0.125 mg, PO, QD
On hand: Digoxin 0.25 mg tablets

Ratio-Proportion

$0.125mg : X\ tab = 0.25mg : 1\ tab$

$0.125mg : X\ tab = 0.25mg : 1\ tab$

$0.25\ X = 0.125$

$\dfrac{0.25\ X}{0.25} = \dfrac{0.125}{0.25}$

$$0.25\overline{)0.125}\quad \dfrac{0.5}{}$$

$$\begin{array}{r} 0 \\ \hline 125 \\ 125 \\ \hline 0 \end{array}$$

$X = 0.5\ tab$

Fraction Method

$\dfrac{0.125mg}{X\ tab} = \dfrac{0.25\ mg}{1\ tab}$

$\dfrac{0.125mg}{X\ tab} \diagup\diagdown \dfrac{0.25\ mg}{1\ tab}$

$0.25\ X = 0.125$

$\dfrac{0.25}{0.25} X = \dfrac{0.125}{0.25}$

$$0.25\overline{)0.125}\quad \dfrac{0.5}{}$$

$$\begin{array}{r} 0 \\ \hline 125 \\ 125 \\ \hline 0 \end{array}$$

$X = 0.5\ tab$

Desired over Have

$\dfrac{0.125mg}{0.25\ mg} \times 1\ tab =$

$\dfrac{0.125mg}{0.25mg} \times 1\ tab = \dfrac{0.125}{0.25}\ tab$

$$0.25\overline{)0.125} = 0.5\ tab\quad \dfrac{0.5}{}$$

$$\begin{array}{r} 0 \\ \hline 125 \\ 125 \\ \hline 0 \end{array}$$

Dimensional Analysis

$0.125\ mg \times \dfrac{\quad\quad}{mg} =$

$0.125mg \times \dfrac{1\ tab}{0.25\ mg} = \dfrac{0.125}{0.25}\ tab$

$$0.25\overline{)0.125} = 0.5\ tab\quad \dfrac{0.5}{}$$

$$\begin{array}{r} 0 \\ \hline 125 \\ 125 \\ \hline 0 \end{array}$$

Practice all Four Question Seven Answer

Ordered: Synthroid 50 mcg, PO, QD
On hand: Synthroid 0.025 mg tablets

Ratio-Proportion

$50\,mcg : X\,mg = 1000\,mcg = 1\,mg$

$50\,mcg : X\,mg = 1000\,mcg : 1\,mg$

$1000\,X = 50$

$\dfrac{1000}{1000}\,X = \dfrac{50}{1000}$

$X = $ $1000\,\overline{)50.00}$ $\;\;.05$
$\underline{0}$
5000
$\underline{5000}$
0

$X = 0.05\,mg$

$0.05\,mg : X\,tab = 0.025\,mg : 1\,tab$

$0.05\,mg : X\,tab = 0.025\,mg : 1\,tab$

$0.025\,X = 0.05$

$\dfrac{0.025\,X}{0.025} = \dfrac{0.05}{0.025}$

$X = $ $0.025\,\overline{)0.050}$ $\;\;2.$
$\underline{50}$
0

$X = 2\,tabs$

Fraction Method

$$\frac{50\,mcg}{X\,mg} = \frac{1000\,mcg}{1\,mg}$$

$$\frac{50\,mcg}{X\,mg} \diagup\!\!\!\!\diagdown \frac{1000\,mcg}{1\,mg}$$

$$1000\,X = 50$$

$$\frac{1000}{1000}X = \frac{50}{1000}$$

$$X = \quad 1000\overline{)50.00} \quad \begin{array}{r} .05 \\ \hline 0 \\ 5000 \\ 5000 \\ \hline 0 \end{array}$$

$$X = 0.05\,mg$$

$$\frac{0.05\,mg}{X\,tab} = \frac{0.025\,mg}{1\,tab}$$

$$\frac{0.05\,mg}{X\,tab} \diagup\!\!\!\!\diagdown \frac{0.025\,mg}{1\,tab}$$

$$0.025\,X = 0.05$$

$$\frac{0.025\,X}{0.025} = \frac{0.05}{0.025}$$

$$X = \quad 0.025\overline{)0.050} \quad \begin{array}{r} 2. \\ \hline 50 \\ 50 \\ \hline 0 \end{array}$$

$$X = 2\,tabs$$

Desired over Have

$$\frac{50 \text{ mcg}}{1000 \text{ mcg}} \times 1 \text{ mg} \ =$$

$$\frac{50 \text{ mcg}}{1000 \text{ mcg}} \times 1 \text{ mg} \ = \frac{50}{1000} \text{ mg}$$

$$1000 \overline{\smash{)}\,50.00} \ \ ^{.05} \ = 0.05 \text{ mg}$$
$$\frac{5000}{5000}$$
$$\frac{5000}{0}$$

$$\frac{0.05 \text{ mg}}{0.025 \text{ mg}} \times 1 \text{ tab} \ =$$

$$\frac{0.05 \text{ mg}}{0.025 \text{ mg}} \times 1 \text{ tab} \ = \frac{0.05}{0.025} \text{ tab}$$

$$0.025 \overline{\smash{)}\,0.050} \ \ ^{2.} \ = 2 \text{ tabs}$$
$$\frac{50}{0}$$

Dimensional Analysis

$$50 \text{ mcg} \times \frac{\ \ \ }{\text{mcg}} \times \underline{\ \ \ } \ =$$

$$50 \text{ mcg} \times \frac{1 \text{ mg}}{1000 \text{ mcg}} \times \frac{\ \ \ }{\text{mg}} \ =$$

$$50 \text{ mcg} \times \frac{1 \text{ mg}}{1000 \text{ mcg}} \times \frac{1 \text{ tab}}{0.025 \text{ mg}} \ =$$

$$50 \text{ mcg} \times \frac{1 \text{ mg}}{1000 \text{ mcg}} \times \frac{1 \text{ tab}}{0.025 \text{ mg}} \ = \frac{50}{25} \text{ tab}$$

$$= 2 \text{ tab}$$

Practice all Four Question Eight Answer

Ordered: Atropine gr 1/150 , IM, on call to OR
On hand: Atropine 0.4 mg / ml

Ratio-Proportion

$$gr \frac{1}{150} : X mg = gr 1 : 60 mg$$

$$gr \frac{1}{150} : X mg = gr 1 : 60 mg$$

$$X = \frac{1}{150} \times 60$$

$$X = \frac{60}{150}$$

$$150 \overline{)\,60.0\,} \;\; .4$$
$$\underline{60\ 0}$$
$$0$$

$$X = 0.4 \; mg$$

Fraction Method

$$\frac{gr \frac{1}{150}}{X mg} = \frac{gr 1}{60 mg}$$

$$\frac{gr \frac{1}{150}}{X mg} \diagdown \frac{gr 1}{60 mg}$$

$$X = \frac{1}{150} \times 60$$

$$X = \frac{60}{150} \qquad 150 \overline{)\,60.0\,} \;\; .4$$
$$\underline{60\ 0}$$
$$0$$

$$X = 0.4 mg$$

Desired over Have

$$\frac{gr \frac{1}{150} \times \frac{60 mg}{gr 1}}{} =$$

$$\frac{gr \frac{1}{150} \times 60 mg}{gr 1} = \frac{1}{150} \times 60 = \frac{60}{150} mg$$

$$150 \overline{)\,60.0\,} \;\; .4 = 0.4 mg$$
$$\underline{60\ 0}$$
$$0$$

72

Dimensional Analysis

$$gr \frac{1}{150} \times \frac{}{gr} \times \frac{}{} =$$

$$gr \frac{1}{150} \times \frac{60 \, mg}{gr \; 1} \times \frac{}{mg} =$$

$$gr \frac{1}{150} \times \frac{60 \, mg}{gr \; 1} \times \frac{1 \, ml}{0.4 \, mg} = \frac{\frac{60}{150}}{0.4} \, ml = \frac{0.4}{0.4} \, ml$$

$$= 1 \, ml$$

Practice all Four Question Nine Answer

Ordered: Acetazolamide 1gm, PO, Now
On hand: Acetazolamide 500 mg tablets

Ratio-Proportion

$$1gm : X mg : 1gm : 1000mg$$

Same as conversion so no
calculation need to do the
conversion

$$1 gm = 1000mg$$

$$1000mg : X tab = 500 mg : 1 tab$$

$$1000 mg : X tab = 500 mg : 1 tab$$

$$500 X = 1000$$

$$\frac{500}{500} X = \frac{1000}{500}$$

$$X = 2 \ tab$$

Fraction Method

$$\frac{1gm}{X mg} = \frac{1 gm}{1000 mg}$$

Same as conversion factor
So no calculation needed to
do the conversion

$$1gm = 1000 mg$$

$$\frac{1000mg}{X tab} = \frac{500mg}{1 tab}$$

$$\frac{1000 mg}{X tab} \diagdown \frac{500 mg}{1 tab}$$

$$500 X = 1000$$

$$\frac{500}{500} X = \frac{1000}{500}$$

$$X = 2 \ tabs$$

Desired over Have

$$\frac{1gm}{1 gm} \times 1000 \ mg = 1000mg$$

$$\frac{1000 mg}{500 mg} \times 1 tab = \frac{1000}{500} \ tab$$

$$= 2 \ tabs$$

Dimensional Analysis

$$1 \text{ gm} \times \frac{}{\text{gm}} \times \frac{}{} =$$

$$1 \text{ gm} \times \frac{1000 \text{ mg}}{1 \text{ gm}} \times \frac{}{\text{mg}} =$$

$$1 \text{ gm} \times \frac{1000 \text{ mg}}{1 \text{ gm}} \times \frac{1 \text{ tab}}{500 \text{ mg}} =$$

$$1 \text{ gm} \times \frac{1000 \text{ mg}}{1 \text{ gm}} \times \frac{1 \text{ tab}}{500 \text{ mg}} = \frac{1000}{500} \text{ tab}$$

$$= 2 \text{ tabs}$$

Practice all Four Question Ten Answer

Ordered: Heparin 5000 units, SQ, Q12h
On hand: Heparin 10,000 units / ml

Ratio-Proportion

$$5000 \text{ units} : X\,ml = 10,000 \text{ units} : 1\,ml$$

$$5000 \text{ units} : X\,ml = 10,000 \text{ units} : 1\,ml$$

$$10,000\,X = 5000$$

$$\frac{10\,000}{10000}X = \frac{5000}{10000}$$

$$X = \frac{1}{2}\,ml$$

Fraction Method

$$\frac{5000 \text{ units}}{X\,ml} = \frac{10,000 \text{ units}}{1\,ml}$$

$$\frac{5000 \text{ units}}{X\,ml} \diagup \frac{10,000 \text{ units}}{1\,ml}$$

$$10,000\,X = 5000$$

$$\frac{10000}{10000}X = \frac{5000}{10000}$$

$$X = \frac{1}{2}\,ml$$

Desired over Have

$$\frac{5000 \text{ units}}{10000 \text{ units}} \times 1\,ml =$$

$$\frac{5000 \text{ units}}{10000 \text{ units}} \times 1\,ml = \frac{5}{10}\,ml$$

$$= \frac{1}{2}\,ml$$

Dimensional Analysis

$$5000 \text{ units} \times \underline{\quad\quad\quad} =$$
$$\text{units}$$

$$5000 \text{ units} \times \frac{1\,ml}{10,000 \text{ units}} = \frac{5000}{10000}\,ml$$

$$\frac{5000}{10000} = \frac{1}{2}\,ml$$

Reconstitution Example Answer

Ratio-Proportion

$250\,mg : \underline{X\,ml} = 500\,mg : \underline{1\,ml}$

$250\,mg : X\,ml = 500\,mg : 1\,ml$

$500x = 250$

$\dfrac{500x}{500} = \dfrac{250}{500}$

$X = \dfrac{1}{2}\,ml$

Fraction Method

$\dfrac{250\,mg}{X\,ml} = \dfrac{500\,mg}{1\,ml}$

$500x = 250$

$\dfrac{500}{500}x = \dfrac{250}{500}$

$X = \dfrac{1}{2}\,ml$

Desired over Have

$\dfrac{250\,mg}{500\,mg} \times 1\,ml =$

$\dfrac{250\,mg}{500\,mg} \times 1\,ml = \dfrac{250}{500}\,ml$

$= \dfrac{1}{2}\,ml$

Dimensional Analysis

$250\,mg \times \dfrac{1\,ml}{500\,mg} =$

$250\,mg \times \dfrac{1\,ml}{500\,mg} = \dfrac{250}{500}\,ml$

$= \dfrac{1}{2}\,ml$

Weight based Example Answer

Ratio-Proportion

$44 \text{ lbs} : X \text{ kg} = 2.2 \text{ lbs} : 1 \text{ kg}$

$44 \text{ lbs} : X \text{ kg} = 2.2 \text{ lbs} : 1 \text{ kg}$

$2.2X = 44$

$\dfrac{2.2}{2.2}X = \dfrac{44}{2.2}$

$X = 2.2\overline{)44.0}$

$X = 20 \text{ kg}$

First find the weight in Kg

$20 \text{ kg} : X \text{ mg} = 1 \text{ kg} : 10 \text{ mg}$ or $20 \times 10 = 200 \text{ mg}$

$X = 200 \text{ mg}$

Now find out what the dose is for the patient weighing 20 kg

$200 \text{ mg} : X \text{ ml} = 100 \text{ mg} : 5 \text{ ml}$

$100X = 1000$

$\dfrac{100}{100}X = \dfrac{1000}{100}$

$X = 10 \text{ ml}$

Now figure out how much you will give the patient

Fraction Method

$\dfrac{44 \text{ lbs}}{X \text{ kg}} = \dfrac{2.2 \text{ lbs}}{1 \text{ kg}}$

$\dfrac{44 \text{ lbs}}{X \text{ kg}} \diagup\!\!\!\!\diagup \dfrac{2.2 \text{ lbs}}{1 \text{ kg}}$

$2.2X = 44$

$\dfrac{2.2}{2.2}X = \dfrac{44}{2.2}$

$X = 2.2\overline{)44.0}$

$X = 20 \text{ kg}$

Use your formula to convert the weight to kg

$\dfrac{20 \text{ kg}}{X \text{ mg}} \diagup\!\!\!\!\diagup \dfrac{1 \text{ kg}}{10 \text{ mg}}$

$X = 200 \text{ mg}$

Now find the dose for the patient for that weight. You could just multiply the weight in kg times 10 but if you want you can use your formula

$\dfrac{200 \text{ mg}}{X \text{ ml}} \diagup\!\!\!\!\diagup \dfrac{100 \text{ mg}}{5 \text{ ml}}$

$100X = 1000$

$\dfrac{100}{100}X = \dfrac{1000}{100}$

$X = 10 \text{ ml}$

Last use your formula again to find the amount to give to the patient

Desired over Have

$$\frac{44 \text{ lbs}}{2.2 \text{ lbs}} \times 1 \text{ kg} =$$

$$\frac{44 \text{ lbs}}{2.2 \text{ lbs}} \times 1 \text{ kg} = \frac{44}{2.2} \text{ kg}$$

$$2.2 \overline{\smash)44.0} \quad \begin{array}{c} 20. \\ \underline{44} \\ 0 \end{array} = 20 \text{ kg}$$

$$\frac{20 \text{ kg}}{1 \text{ kg}} \times 10 \text{ mg} = 200 \text{ mg}$$

$$\frac{200 \text{ mg}}{100 \text{ mg}} \times 5 \text{ ml} =$$

$$\frac{200 \text{ mg}}{100 \text{ mg}} \times 5 \text{ ml} = 10 \text{ ml}$$

Use your formula to convert the weight to kg

Now find the dose for the patient for that weight. You could just multiply the weight in kg times 10 but if you want you can use your formula

Last use your formula again to find the amount to give to the patient

Dimensional Analysis

$$44 \text{ lbs} \times \frac{}{\text{lbs}} \times \frac{}{} \times \frac{}{} =$$

$$44 \text{ lbs} \times \frac{1 \text{ kg}}{2.2 \text{ lbs}} \times \frac{}{\text{kg}} \times \frac{}{} =$$

$$44 \text{ lbs} \times \frac{1 \text{ kg}}{2.2 \text{ lbs}} \times \frac{10 \text{ mg}}{1 \text{ kg}} \times \frac{}{\text{mg}} =$$

$$44 \text{ lbs} \times \frac{1 \text{ kg}}{2.2 \text{ lbs}} \times \frac{10 \text{ mg}}{1 \text{ kg}} \times \frac{5 \text{ ml}}{100 \text{ mg}} =$$

$$44 \text{ lbs} \times \frac{1 \text{ kg}}{2.2 \text{ lbs}} \times \frac{10 \text{ mg}}{1 \text{ kg}} \times \frac{5 \text{ ml}}{100 \text{ mg}} = \frac{2200}{220} \text{ ml}$$

$$= 10 \text{ ml}$$

With dimensional analysis you can add an extra column and convert the weight as well as the dose. With questions like these it is important to always start with what is most specific to the patient. In this case weight. Then use the qualifiers to help you figure out what comes next.

79

Mixing Medications Example Answer

Ratio-Proportion

$20mg : X ml = 50mg : 1ml$

$$50x = 20$$

$$\frac{50}{50}x = \frac{20}{50}$$

$$x = 0.4 ml$$

$10 mg : X ml = 25mg : 1ml$

$$25x = 10$$

$$\frac{25}{25}x = \frac{10}{25}$$

$$X = 0.4 ml$$

Total injection volume   0.8 ml

Fraction Method

$$\frac{20mg}{X ml} \diagup\diagdown \frac{50mg}{1ml}$$

$$50x = 20$$

$$\frac{50x}{50} = \frac{20}{50}$$

$$X = 0.4ml$$

$$\frac{10mg}{X ml} \diagup\diagdown \frac{25mg}{1ml}$$

$$25x = 10$$

$$\frac{25}{25}X = \frac{10}{25}$$

$$X = 0.4 ml$$

total injection volume 0.8ml

Desired over Have

$$\frac{20mg}{50mg} \times 1 ml =$$

$$\frac{20mg}{50mg} \times 1ml = \frac{2}{5}ml$$

$$= 0.4ml$$

$$\frac{10mg}{25mg} \times 1 ml =$$

$$\frac{10mg}{25mg} \times 1ml = \frac{10}{25}ml$$

$$= 0.4ml$$

Total injection volume 0.8ml

Dimensional Analysis

$$20mg \times \frac{1ml}{50mg} = \frac{20}{50}ml$$

$$= 0.4 ml$$

$$10mg \times \frac{1ml}{25mg} = \frac{10}{25}ml$$

$$= 0.4ml$$

total injection volume 0.8 ml

Continuous Infusion Practice Answers

Question 1

Ratio Proportion

1400 units : Xml = 25,000 units : 250 ml

$$25,000 X = 350,000$$

$$\frac{25,000 X}{25,000} = \frac{350,000}{25,000}$$

$$X = 25\overline{)350}^{\,14}$$
$$\quad\quad \underline{25}$$
$$\quad\quad 100$$

$$X = 14 \text{ ml/hr}$$

Fraction Method

$$\frac{1400 \text{ units}}{Xml} \diagup\!\!\!\!\diagdown \frac{25000}{250}$$

$$25,000 x = 350,000$$

$$\frac{25,000}{25,000} X = \frac{350,000}{25,000}$$

$$X = 14 \text{ ml/hr}$$

Desired over have

$$\frac{1400 \text{ units}}{25,000 \text{ units}} \times 250 ml =$$

$$\frac{1400 \text{ units}}{25,000 \text{ units}} \times 250 ml = \frac{350,000}{25,000}$$

$$= 14 ml/hr$$

Dimensional Analysis

$$1400 \text{ units} \times \frac{250 ml}{25,000 \text{ units}} =$$

$$1400 \text{ units} \times \frac{250 ml}{25,000 \text{ units}} = \frac{350,000}{25,000}$$

$$= 14 ml/hr$$

Question 2

Ratio Proportion

$16\text{ml} : X \text{ units} = 500\text{ml} : 25000 \text{ units}$

$$500x = 400,000$$

$$\frac{500x}{500} = \frac{400,000}{500}$$

$$\begin{array}{r} 800 \\ 5\overline{\smash)4000} \\ \underline{40} \\ 0 \end{array}$$

$$X = 800 \text{ units}/hr$$

Fraction Method

$$\frac{16\text{ml}}{X \text{ units}} \times \frac{500\text{ml}}{25,000 \text{ units}}$$

$$500 \text{ units} = 400,000$$

$$\frac{500}{500}x = \frac{400,000}{500}$$

$$x = 800 \text{ units}/hr$$

Desired over have

$$\frac{16\text{ml}}{500 \text{ ml}} \times 25,000 \text{ units} =$$

$$\frac{16\text{ml}}{500 \text{ ml}} \times 25,000 \text{ units} = \frac{400,000}{500} \text{ units}$$

$$= 800 \text{ units}/hr$$

Dimensional Analysis

$$16\text{ ml} \times \frac{25000 \text{ units}}{500 \text{ ml}} =$$

$$16\text{ ml} \times \frac{25,000 \text{ units}}{500 \text{ ml}} = \frac{4000}{5} \text{ units}$$

$$= 800 \text{ units}/hr$$

82

Question 3

$15ml : Xmg = 250ml : 500mg$

$250x = 7500$

$\dfrac{250}{250}x = \dfrac{7500}{250}$

$$25\overline{\smash{\big)}750}$$
$$\underline{75}$$
$$0$$

quotient: 30

$X = 30\,mg/hr$

Fraction Method

$\dfrac{15ml}{Xmg} \diagdown\!\!\!\!\diagup \dfrac{250ml}{500mg}$

$250X = 7500$

$\dfrac{250}{250}X = \dfrac{7500}{250}$

$X = 30\,mg/hr$

Desired over have

$\dfrac{15ml}{250ml} \times 500mg =$

$\dfrac{15ml}{250ml} \times 500mg = \dfrac{7500}{250}mg$

$= 30\,mg/hr$

Dimensional Analysis

$15ml \times \dfrac{500mg}{250ml} =$

$15ml \times \dfrac{500mg}{250ml} = \dfrac{7500}{250}mg$

$= 30\,mg/hr$

83

Extra Math Scaffold

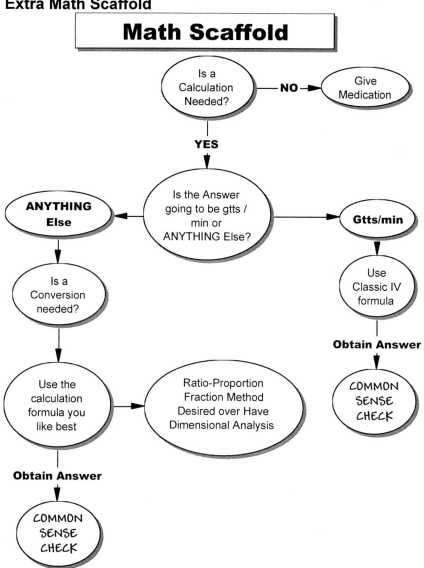

Math Scaffold

Is a Calculation Needed? — **NO** → Give Medication

YES

Is the Answer going to be gtts / min or ANYTHING Else?

ANYTHING Else

Gtts/min

Is a Conversion needed?

Use Classic IV formula

Use the calculation formula you like best

Ratio-Proportion Fraction Method Desired over Have Dimensional Analysis

Obtain Answer

COMMON SENSE CHECK

Obtain Answer

COMMON SENSE CHECK

Extra conversion equivalents

Metric

1000 grams	= 1 Kilogram
1000 milligrams	= 1 gram
1000 micrograms	= 1 milligram
1000 milliliter	= 1 Liter

Equivalents between Systems

1 Kilogram	= 2.2 pounds
1 grain	= 60 mg (some texts say 62.5 or 65 there is a 10% leeway)
1 fluid ounce	= 30ml
1 cup = 8 ounces	= 240 mlliliters
1 teaspoon	= 5 milliliters
1 tablespoon	= 15 mlliliters

85

Epilogue

If you have made it this far you should be ready to tackle any basic pharmacology math test that comes your way. With determination, persistence, and practice you will not be conquered by pharmacology math. If you have questions contact me at Karen@nursethings.com. I stand by my methods and will do my best to help you if you feel this book has not.

Also Available from Nursethings

For Students:

Nursing Notes the Easy Way:100+ Common Nursing Documentation and Communication Templates
Ever wonder what to put in a nursing note? Not sure what to say when giving report or calling the physician? This pocket- sized guide provides you with over a hundred templates for written and verbal communications so you will never be at a loss for words. (18.00)

Survival Tips for the Nursing Student in Adult Med-Surg Clinical
Indispensable for success in clinical! This pocket-sized guide provides the common questions clinical instructors ask students about various conditions, labs, and medication administration and how to answer them. Also includes preparing for clinical, how to review the chart quickly, quick lab evaluation, and how to give report. Need to do a procedure or give a medication? This guide will provide you with an equipment list and steps to take. Written by nursing instructors with a combined 25 years of clinical instruction (Man, we're getting old!) (24.00)

On-Campus Uniform Polo shirts and other apparel

For Faculty:

Nursing Education STAT : Rx for Student Success
Especially for Nursing Faculty, this practical, concise guide will assist you in working with students experiencing difficulty or help those "B" students take it to the next level. Techniques are presented for ease of immediate application. ($28.00)

Nursing Education STAT: What they didn't' tell you in orientation, A survival guide for clinical Instructors
Especially made for clinical instructors, this guide will help you understand everything from navigating your educational institution to counseling students for poor performance. Includes instructor insights and the student content from Survival Tips for the Nursing Student in Adult Med-Surg Clinicals.

All of our products are available to use as fundraising items!!

www.NURSETHINGS.com